# FROM LESION TO METAPHOR: CHRONIC PAIN IN BRITISH, FRENCH AND GERMAN MEDICAL WRITINGS, 1800–1914

Andrew Hodgkiss

Amsterdam – Atlanta, GA 2000

First published in 2000
by Editions Rodopi B. V., Amsterdam – Atlanta, GA 2000.

Hodgkiss, Andrew © 2000

Design and Typesetting by Alex Mayor, the Wellcome Trust.
Printed and bound in The Netherlands by Editions Rodopi B. V.,
Amsterdam – Atlanta, GA 2000.

**British Library Cataloguing in Publication Data**
A catalogue record for this book is available from the British
Library
ISBN: 90-420-0821-0 (Paper)
ISBN: 90-420-0831-8 (Bound)

From Lesion to Metaphor: Chronic Pain in British, French and
German Medical Writings: 1800–1914 –
Amsterdam – Atlanta, GA:
Rodopi. – ill.
(Clio Medica 58 / ISSN 0045-7183;
The Wellcome Institute Series in the History of Medicine)

Front cover:
Cover design is a collage of portraits of Bichat, Wittgenstein and Freud.
Reproduced by kind permission of the Wellcome Trust, the Library of
Trinity College, Cambridge. Freud image: © Freud Museum.

© Editions Rodopi B. V., Amsterdam – Atlanta, GA 2000

Printed in The Netherlands

All titles in the Clio Medica series (from 1999 onwards) are available to
download from the CatchWord website: http://www.catchword.co.uk

# Contents

# Abstract

This is the first monograph devoted to the history of chronic pain. A novel methodology is used. Examining responses to a problem that remained stable over time anchors a survey of shifting terms and theories and leaves the historical invariance of the clinical syndrome open to textual research. Writings by medical authors from a wide range of professional backgrounds are examined including surgeons, physicians, psychiatrists, neurophysiologists, neurologists and psychoanalysts.

Early responses to the problem of chronic pain without structural lesion were the appearance of neuralgia, a neuro-anatomical rewriting of traditional sympathies, extension of the concept of lesion to embrace disturbance of function and appeals to cenesthesis. Later in the century distinctions were drawn between hysterical and neuralgic pain, and between ideogenic, psychogenic and neurogenic pain. Some argued for the physiological equivalence of chronic pain and melancholia, while pain was central to Freud's original notion of conversion.

This evidence of continuous discussion of lesionless pain throughout the century challenges the orthodox historical view that the rise of neuroscience meant such pain was simply dismissed as imaginary. The historical invariance of a syndrome of chronic pain without lesion speaks against histories of lesionless syndromes premised on social constructionism. The historical findings are relevant to contemporary debates about the nosology and nature of chronic pain.

# Acknowledgements

I should like to thank Professor J. P. Watson at the Division of Psychiatry and Psychology, King's College London at Guy's Hospital, for nurturing the early signs of my interest in pain and for supporting my research interests in the psychiatric humanities since 1985. Dr G. E. Berrios helped me select this project in 1987 and has offered me a number of important intellectual opportunities since.

Latterly it has been the wonderful academic environment at the Wellcome Institute for the History of Medicine that has accelerated and improved my historical writing. I must single out Professor W. F. Bynum for formal supervision, and Professor R. Porter, Dr S. Jacyna, Professor S. Lawrence and Mr S. Shamdasani for valuable informal discussion. Dr B. Bryan kindly translated passages by Wilhelm Erb and Otto Binswanger from the German.

The neuroses and psychoanalysis are not high on the agenda of many psychiatric academics or clinicians in London at present, in stark contrast to Paris. My thinking on these subjects has been enriched through contact with the Centre for Freudian Analysis and Research. Dr B. Benvenuto, Ms D. Machado and Dr R. Klein have particularly influenced me.

The librarians at the Wellcome Institute, the Institute of Neurology, the Royal College of Psychiatrists and the Royal College of Physicians were all most helpful. The friendship and example of Drs J. Coe, J. May, R. Pite and P. Singer gave me the confidence to attempt this book.

My wife, Dr Stephanie May, and children, Amy and Charles, have loved me and this has made sustained academic work possible.

This research was supported by a one year Medical Graduate Student Fellowship at the Wellcome Institute for the History of Medicine, London. I am most grateful to the Wellcome Trust for funding this in full.

# Introduction

All medical undergraduates are taught something about the distinctions between illness and disease. Illness involves the experience and evaluation of symptoms while disease can be defined as the presence of a lesion. The lesion may be structural or functional. Structural lesions may be obvious on bedside examination or investigative technology may be required to reveal them. Functional lesions are even trickier. Some well-characterized, or at least potentially demonstrable, pathophysiological process is implied. Canguilhem[1] has drawn attention to the difference between dysfunction and hypo- or hyper-function in this context. The former is a qualitative variation from normal physiology while the latter is a quantitative variation.

It is interesting to note that being ill is largely a decision made by the patient, though a doctor may try to challenge the patient's description or evaluation of their experiences and block entry to the sick role.[2, 3] In contrast, judgements about the presence or absence of lesion, and hence disease, are entirely the preserve of doctors and are the cornerstone of their professional hegemony. This is reflected in the priorities of clinical practice. A doctor will be forgiven for misdiagnosing illness but errors concerning disease are considered much more serious. Failure to appreciate that a complaint of headache is to do with concerns about dying of a stroke like father is regarded as a rather minor mistake compared to missing a brain tumour. This, despite the fact that many more lives are blighted by inappropriate long-term analgesic prescribing than by late diagnosis of brain tumours. The priorities of the medical practitioner in this instance are driven by the claims of the profession to exclusive expertise in the diagnosis of disease rather than by epidemiological considerations.

What is not emphasized to medical students is that the distinction between illness and disease described above has only a two hundred year history. Prior to about 1800, physicians in Northern Europe did not think in terms of lesions or claim disease as their area of expertise. Rather they practised medicine at the level of symptoms and syndromes, classifying them by surface characteristics in

1

taxonomies based on botanical work. The historian who has made most of this discontinuity in the foundations of medical thought is Michel Foucault (who was actually taught by Canguilhem). In *The Birth of the Clinic*[4] he argued that in France around 1800 there was a revolution in medical ideas. A novel clinical method was developed in which physical signs and post mortem findings became of much greater importance than symptoms in medical diagnostics. Foucault introduced the term 'medical gaze' to indicate this shift from a reliance on the patient's words to examination of his body. He went on to argue that a transformation in the power relations between doctor and patient was at stake here. From being servants of the eighteenth-century French gentility, physicians in public hospitals began to see large groups of poor patients as research fodder. Patients offered their bodies as objects for the medical gaze at the cost of respect for their subjectivity. The question 'What seems to be the matter?', which invited a detailed idiosyncratic report of the patient's experience and beliefs, was replaced by 'Where does it hurt?'. This latter enquiry revealed the physician's new assumption that a localized lesion was responsible for the pain and that the patient's self-report, though probably unreliable, might at least direct the examining physician to the relevant part of the body.

The above is a summary of some of the ways in which Foucault characterized the 'Paris bedside medicine' that students are still taught in British clinical schools. I was particularly struck by the fact that pain, as a marker of localized tissue lesion, was the exemplar of this clinical method. It occurred to me that pain without any lesion must have constituted a major difficulty for nineteenth-century physicians adopting such a praxis. Most historians commenting on this have suggested that after the early 1800s lesionless pain was regarded as 'imaginary', not a real pain at all.[5, 6, 7] They further argue that subsequent neuroscientific research, elucidating a 'pain pathway' in the nervous system and 'pain spots' in the skin, added more weight to the view that all real pain must have a localizable physical correlate in the body. Their history ends in the early 1960s with the rediscovery of the forgotten insight that pain may be an emotion as much as a sensation, and thus lack an object without being unreal, feigned or imagined. I was suspicious of this cursory historical argument and decided to study the history of pain without lesion in nineteenth-century medical writings in detail.

Why is research on a lesionless symptom by a doctor worthwhile, given that such symptoms do not arise from 'real' disease and are not life-threatening? The first, and in my view most important, answer is that this phenomenon is common, especially in primary care settings. It lies at the limit, and reveals the limitations, of the clinical method we still employ. Secondly, chronic symptoms without lesions, such as pain and fatigue, can be extremely disabling and cause much suffering. I am not the first to write a history of a lesionless symptom: Wessely[8] and Shorter[9] have done so already. But this book is, I believe, the first to highlight the unique challenge that lesionless pain represented to clinical method after 1800. Pain, which was supposed to be the marker of a spatially localized structural lesion, posed a greater threat to the claims of the new 'anatomoclinical' method when unaccompanied by lesion than did more diffuse lesionless symptoms such as fatigue.

There are a good many other reasons why pain without lesion has been chosen as a topic here. Psychiatrists remain in a conceptual and nosological quandary about the phenomenon, sometimes employing terms such as Somatoform Pain Disorder as a mere diagnosis of exclusion (in DSM III-R[10]; see Murphy[11] for a fuller critique), more recently insisting on psychogenesis of the pain yet setting it apart from conversion disorder and mood disorders (Pain Disorder in DSM IV[12]). I hope my research will contribute to this field. There is growing interest in pain as a medical specialty in its own right with the proliferation of pain clinics in the United States, France and the United Kingdom and the management of chronic pain is central to the developing sub-specialty of liaison psychiatry. Within academic history of medicine there is an increasing interest in trying to include the experience of patients, especially of their bodies, in historical research. And, finally, because pain has a special place in the thought of two of the most brilliant intellectuals of our own century, namely Ludwig Wittgenstein and Michel Foucault. It seems to me to be lamentable that their writings on pain have made so little impact on medical practitioners to date. This book is, in part, an attempt to start to address this.

Although Wittgenstein will not be specifically mentioned again, my continuing encounter with his comments on pain in *Philosophical Investigations*[13] has guided both choice and treatment of this topic. The lengthy quotation below raises a series of issues about the incorrigibility of pain reports, pain and subjectivity, pain localization and the relationship between pain and language. A useful introduction to some of the philosophical aspects of pain has been provided by Smith & Jones.[14] They elaborate distinctions between causal, phenomenological and functionalist accounts of pain; that is, between pain as a *consequence* of specified causes, as a *lived experience*

3

accessible through introspection and as a *cause* of various pain behaviours. Wittgenstein explored the limitations of each of these positions. Although this book is historical and not philosophical I have tried to draw out these issues in my readings of nineteenth-century medical texts.

> But isn't it absurd to say of a *body* that it has pain? – And why does one feel an absurdity in that? In what sense is it true that my hand does not feel pain, but I in my hand?...if someone has a pain in his hand, then the hand does not say so (unless it writes it) and one does not comfort the hand, but the sufferer: one looks into his face...
>
> Now someone tells me that *he* knows what pain is only from his own case! – Suppose everyone had a box with something in it: we call it a 'beetle'. No one can look into anyone else's box, and everyone says he knows what a beetle is only by looking at *his* beetle. – Here it would be quite possible for everyone to have something different in his box. One might even imagine such a thing constantly changing. – But suppose the word 'beetle' had a use in these people's language? – If so it would not be used as the name of a thing. The thing in the box has no place in the language-game at all; not even as a *something*: for the box might even be empty. – No, one can 'divide through' by the thing in the box; it cancels out, whatever it is.
>
> That is to say: if we construe the grammar of the expression of sensation on the model of 'object and designation' the object drops out of consideration as irrelevant...
>
> 'Yes, but there is *something* there all the same accompanying my cry of pain. And it is on account of that that I utter it. And this something is what is important – and frightful.' – Only whom are we informing of this? And on what occasion?...
>
> Pain–behaviour can point to a painful place – but the subject of pain is the person who gives it expression.[15]

## Notes

1 Canguilhem, 1989, *The Normal and the Pathological.*
2 Mechanic, 1962, *The concept of illness behaviour.*
3 Pilowsky, 1969, *Abnormal illness behaviour.*
4 Foucault, 1973, *The Birth of the Clinic: an archaeology of medical perception.*
5 Merskey & Spear, 1967, *Pain: psychological and psychiatric aspects.*
6 Morris, 1991, *The Culture of Pain.*
7 Rey, 1993, *History of Pain.*
8 Wessely, 1990, *Old wine in new bottles: neurasthenia and 'M.E.'*

9  Shorter, 1992, *From Paralysis to Fatigue: a history of psychosomatic illness in the modern era.*

10  DSM III-R, American Psychiatric Association, 1987.

11  Murphy, 1990, *Classification of the somatoform disorders.*

12  DSM-IV, American Psychiatric Association, 1994.

13  Wittgenstein, 1958, *Philosophical Investigations.*

14  Smith & Jones, 1986, *The Philosophy of Mind.*

15  Wittgenstein, 1958, 98–101, *Philosophical Investigations.*

## Secondary Literature Review
## and Methodological Remarks.

No secondary source is confined entirely to the history of pain without lesion though Merskey & Spear,[1] Morris,[2] and Shorter[3] contain lengthy contributions on the topic. Relevant material is scattered among secondary texts on a range of subjects. Histories of pain, neuralgia and the neuroses have proven most useful. Valuable passages are also available in more general histories of neurology and experimental psychology.

### History of Pain Without Lesion

Merskey & Spear[4] state that neglect of psychological aspects of pain and minimization of the importance of emotion in pain perception 'came easily in the wake of seemingly definitive discoveries in anatomy and physiology' in the second half of the nineteenth century. They single out the work on pain by Charles Bell and Johannes Müller as 'substantial evidence that pain was mediated by specific nerve endings and pathways.' Henceforth 'pains became either real, i.e. due to organic or functional afflictions of the nerves, or else imaginary.'

Several objections to this historical view might be raised initially. Their argument glosses over the complexities of the evolving meaning of the term 'functional' in the nineteenth century, though in a later book Merskey[5] did address this. The extent to which Schiff, Gowers and others conceived a simple relationship between stimuli and pain is overstated. These authors confined themselves to the claim that they were discovering something about the conditions of spinal cord integrity under which pain was and was not felt. They never went so far as to reduce pain to a simple response to a stimulus.[6] Müller's position is definitely misrepresented by Merskey & Spear insofar as he did not regard pain as a sensory modality in its own right, but rather as a qualitative variation of the sense of touch. Thus he never claimed pain had a neuro-anatomical pathway of its own (see Chapters 3 & 4 below). Despite these problems, this short historical overview provides a useful introduction to our topic. It is particularly valuable for emphasizing that early-nineteenth-century British writings on pain without lesion were by surgeons and physicians rather than psychiatrists. This theme, of a history of a psychiatric illness to be found in non-psychiatric clinical settings and texts, will recur throughout my work. Interestingly the current practice of liaison psychiatry involves the detection and treatment of psychiatric conditions in medical and surgical patient populations.

Morris exaggerates Merskey & Spear's argument, lumping together 'Bell, Magendie, Müller, Weber, von Frey and Schiff' as responsible for 'the scientific basis for believing that pain was owing simply to the stimulation of specific nerve pathways'.[7] Their work, he claims, emptied pain of meaning and reduced it to 'no more than an electrical impulse speeding along the nerves'. He credits the pain clinics that have appeared since the 1960s with challenging this traditional misreading of pain. Morris proffers two more subtle arguments. First he suggests that doubting the reality of a complaint of pain only became possible once a 'positivist medicine rejected pain as an emotion in favour of pain as a sensation arising from lesion'.[8] In my view it is not at all clear that pain was thought of as an emotion prior to the mid-nineteenth century. Indeed, the concept of emotion has its own complex history and this undermines Morris's claim. Having said this, it has been suggested that physicians tended to see their own 'objective' judgements about the presence or absence of lesions as more significant and reliable than the mere subjective complaints of patients as a new clinical method was adopted in the early nineteenth century. Foucault[9] and Jewson[10] have argued that the 'medical gaze' reflected and created altered power relations between doctor and patient. The search for visual proof (lesions corresponding to pains) then 'trumped' the patient's speech.

The second argument Morris propounds is that 'hysteria provides important evidence that pain is constructed as much by social conditions as by the structure of the nervous system'.[11] This is a stance known as social constructionism and I think there are a number of reasons to doubt the widely held view that lesionless symptoms, above all other medical conditions, are socially constructed. The 'strong' social constructionist is obliged to demonstrate that pain without lesion varies in quality or in prevalence over time and must offer explanations for this in terms of social factors. If the clinical picture and prevalence of lesionless pain is rather historically invariant, their position falls. We shall see that the left-sided predominance of pain without lesion, the continuous, dull, boring, severe qualities of the pain, the severe disability and opiate-dependence associated with it, are all described time and again in case histories throughout the nineteenth century. There is also evidence in both primary and secondary sources that points to the sustained high prevalence of chronic pain without lesion from 1790 to 1910. The best example is Briquet's work on the epidemiology of hysteria in mid-nineteenth-century French inpatients.[12] He found left-sided pain to be the commonest lesionless symptom. Risse's historical study of the symptoms of hysterics in the Edinburgh Infirmary around 1790[13] reveals the same high prevalence of pains. Historical 'numbers arguments' of this sort can be difficult to resolve but I hope I have said enough to at least put Morris's position into question. By way of an alternative to the social constructionist view, Merskey & Watson[14] have suggested that the historically invariant left-sided predominance of pain without lesion reflects an organic basis for the phenomenon, possibly right hemisphere dominance for emotion.

Shorter's book on the history of somatized symptoms[15] is perhaps closest to my topic of all the secondary literature. While it has proven a rich source of primary materials, I shall not be taking its historical methodology as a guide and most of my conclusions are at odds with Shorter.

The whole notion of writing a history of somatoform disorders or somatized symptoms before 1900 is hopelessly anachronistic if, like Shorter, one defines such symptoms as 'caused by the action of the unconscious mind.'[16] I contend that my approach of asking whether symptom without lesion was recognized, regarded as problematic and, if so, how it was theorized, is methodologically superior. Secondly, even within his own terms, Shorter fails to address the possibility of a distinction between 'psychosomatic' and 'conversion' symptoms that has so exercised psychoanalysts in the twentieth century. Thirdly, he makes extensive use of retrospective diagnosis to pick out somatized symptoms and disorders in nineteenth-century case histories, basing his judgements on rapid recovery with placebo or even by 'the smell' of the case. I have attempted to avoid retrospective diagnoses entirely and to confine myself to the terminology and explanation brought to bear on the problem of lesionless pain at the time. I am well aware that most of the pains that were 'non-lesional' in the early nineteenth century would be regarded as of organic origin in the light of current investigative technology. This is not important for a history of terms or ideas. I shall be attempting to write a history of a clinical conundrum that was both invariant and seen as problematic throughout the chosen period.

Shorter, like Morris, starts from a strong position, arguing for the social construction of all somatized symptoms and syndromes. He assumes that the material available to 'the unconscious' is culturally determined and also, most remarkably, that 'the unconscious mind desires to be taken seriously' in its choice of somatic expression.[17] These factors explain, for him, why somatized symptoms vary over time. Shorter argues that hysterical women stopped displaying astasia-abasia after 1900 because bedside neurological examination improved (with the introduction of Babinski's sign) to such an extent that they risked their symptom not being taken seriously and because the sociocultural position of women altered. There are, in my view, several objections to this line of argument. We are invited to assume the existence of 'the unconscious' as a cunning, intelligent presence, well informed about developing medical theory and practice. In addition, Shorter's account of the social construction of somatized symptoms is unconvincing. It seems a long step from alluding to rich women dressing as flappers, smoking in public and riding motorbikes in the 1920s to the assertion that women of that time were under less pressure to care for elderly relatives or less burdened with childcare than those 30 years before. And an even longer step from there to a new 'choice' of symptom. Surely the whole thrust of the Freudian corpus is that hysterical conversion symptoms are intensely idiosyncratic and rooted in biography rather than socially determined by the zeitgeist of an era? Finally, the evidence I mentioned above, pointing to historical invariance in the quality and prevalence of somatized symptoms, counts against the strong social constructionist position.

Despite these methodological weaknesses, some more detailed explication of Shorter's text is worthwhile. Shorter identifies three early-nineteenth-century conceptual strands as central to his topic: clinicopathological correlation, irritation and reflex theory. The combination of these yielded 'spinal irritation' and the reflex theory of hysteria. Shorter speaks of the 1840s as the 'heyday' of spinal irritation. It fell out of favour in elite medicine after Romberg wrote against it around 1850,[18] but persisted in the spas of Europe until at least 1900.[19] The reflex theory of hysteria is depicted as growing out of Marshall Hall's work, as elaborated by Romberg. Irritation of the internal genital organs of women resulted in motor symptoms of hysteria via a reflex arc involving the nervous system. From 1850 to 1900 this gynaecological theory of hysteria was predominant and a good deal of genital surgery was performed by way of treatment. Shorter gives an interesting reading of Charcot's work on hysteria.[20] He points out that pain without lesion was central to 'local hysteria' and claims that Charcot 'upgraded symptoms on the sensory side' after 1880. Charcot's interest in the psychology of hysteria is depicted as late and minor.

## History of Pain

Perhaps the most straightforward genre in the literature is the history of scientific and medical ideas about the neuro-anatomy and neurophysiology of pain. Two outstanding accounts are available in English: Keele[21] and Rey.[22]

Keele's monograph is organized around famous names in the history of pain, from antiquity to the mid-twentieth-century. Virtually no context is offered in which to place these canonical experiments and authors. What the book lacks in methodological sophistication is outweighed by the lucid summaries of the thought of these various authorities. Concerning my period of interest, 1800 to 1914, there are concise expositions of work on pain by Bichat, Bell, Magendie, Müller, Weber, Brown-Séquard, Schiff, Gowers and von Frey. Keele argues that 'the quest for structural equivalents for each sense' began after Müller had propounded the law of specific nervous energy (i.e. after 1830) and that animal experimentation, as pioneered by Magendie, was the main tool of enquiry.[23] For example, Schiff and Brown-Séquard are described as 'analysing sensory modes within the cord'. By 1886 Gowers could make a seemingly definitive statement: it was 'almost certain that the anterolateral ascending tract constitutes the path for sensibility to pain'.[24] But, Keele points out, Gowers later had doubts and Bechterev explicitly rejected any project of localizing sensory pathways in the cord in 1899.

Keele presents evidence of a nineteenth-century tradition of doubt concerning 'pain pathways', and even about pain's status as a special sense, that ran in parallel with 'the discovery of the spinothalamic tract'. For example, Weber never accepted pain, hunger or thirst as sensory modes because they lacked external referents. He, Erb and Wundt all favoured overstimulation of other sensory nerves, rather than any special neuro-anatomy, as the basis of pain. For these Germans, pain was an alteration in bodily sensation, the *Gemeingefühl,* rather than a sensation of any external object. Keele goes on to take sides. The idea of a 'rigid neural architecture subserving pain', a pain pathway, has, he asserts, proven inadequate to account for the variety of pain seen in clinical practice. Von Frey's 'pain spots' are singled out for special blame here. Keele then points to the early-twentieth-century electrophysiological research on inhibition, selection, summation and integration of nerve impulses as providing a more sophisticated, dynamic model of pain perception.

Finally he turns to the challenge of chronic pain which may be lesionless and non-anatomically distributed: 'perpetuated pain is always complex pain...a pain edifice'. He suggests that non-anatomical pain is localized by 'ideated percepts imposed upon the background of the body image' and that they are confined to 'primitive societies'.[25] 'To understand and to exert influence on such pain it is largely unnecessary to know any physiology, but only the minds of men'. Thus Keele recognizes chronic pain without lesion and asserts that a psychological aetiology is at play, but does not attempt to write its history. Instead he provides a crude anthropology.

Taken as a whole, Keele's book is puzzling. On the one hand he seems keen to draw attention to the complexity of pain and the limitations of an approach based on a 'pathway'. On the other, he dismisses chronic pain without lesion as the province of impressionable 'primitives' and charlatan doctors. This apparent contradiction in his position can be explained. He favours very complex neurophysiological explanations for clinical pain but rejects mere psychological theories. He would have welcomed Melzack & Wall's 'gate theory' of 1965[26] which proposed an influence on pain from descending tracts in the spinal cord. This bias led him to write a partial history which describes the neuroscientific work but omits writings on the psychology of pain. The great value of Keele's story is that it emphasizes that the quest for pain pathways, the reductionist tradition, was shadowed by an alternative school in Germany for whom pain was a dimension of the *Gemeingefühl*, not a sensation proper at all, and lacked any special neuro-anatomy. This crucial point immediately puts in question the consensus view of Merskey & Spear,[27] Morris[28] and Rey[29] that pain reductionism silenced consideration of psychological aspects of pain in the nineteenth-century.

Rey's more recent, and rather longer, book[30] covers similar ground but is more historically sophisticated, providing context and offering historical explanations for changing ideas. She argues that the secularization of pain in the eighteenth century, through Protestantism and 'the creation of the individual' in the Enlightenment, was a crucial prerequisite for any scientific study of pain. The theological links with Original Sin and Christ's Passion had to be dismantled before pain could be seen physiologically or even as a personal experience. Another important eighteenth-century development was the definition and measurement of *sensibilité*. She cites Condillac's sensualism as a philosophical precondition for medical reflection on sensibility but argues that 'sensibility was a physiological concept before it was a psychological or aesthetic one'. Mullan,[31] incidentally, has suggested the reverse. Rey points to the work of von Haller and the Montpellier Vitalists in support of her position.

Rey follows Foucault[32] in making much of the discontinuity in medical ideas around 1800. She describes how Bichat used pain as his 'tool of analysis' in distinguishing one tissue from another. Thereafter organ localization, largely unchanged since Galen's *De Locis Affectis*, was replaced by localization at the level of tissues as described in Bichat's *Anatomie Générale* of 1801.[33] She describes how physicians became more impressed by appearance (physical signs) than by speech (symptoms) and how the patient's word was 'continually viewed with suspicion'.[34]

Rey goes on to state that while 'medical texts from the first quarter of the nineteenth century seemed to pay a great deal of attention to the links between "physical" and "mental"',[35] the influence of personal history and mood on pain had later become neglected in the face of advances in neuroscience. In fact 'thinking remained within the global framework of a "specificity theory" throughout the whole nineteenth century, from Johannes Müller to von Frey'.[36] So Rey follows Merskey & Spear[37] and Morris[38] in arguing that reductionist neuroscience obliterated appreciation of psychological aspects of pain. She suggests that this can be explained in the French context by the unhelpful professional distance between experimental neurophysiologists, who followed Magendie and researched *physiological* pain, and clinicians who encountered the messy reality of *pathological* pain. There follow sections describing and commenting in detail on the work of Bell, Magendie, Müller, Bernard, Brown-Séquard and von Frey. I shall allude to these passages in the body of this book.

## History of Neuralgia

Rey warns 'Few painful symptoms have led to so many contradictory interpretations as did neuralgia in the nineteenth century.'[39] She argues that it was a new diagnosis made possible by the spatial localization at tissue level of the new clinical method. At the beginning of the century 'neuralgia' meant pain localized to the course of a nerve but without an inflammatory structural lesion.[40] The criteria of this definition would have been meaningless prior to Bichat's work. The term was actually coined by Chaussier in 1802. Rey explains how, from the outset

> neuralgia was caught between two interpretations, one which
> wanted to identify it as being due to transient inflammation of

unknown causes even though this did not agree with most observations, and the other which, in view of the failure of pathological anatomy to find any lesions, was likely to identify it as [a neurosis].[41]

The debate raged for decades.

Alam & Merskey[42] have written a comprehensive overview of the changing referent of the term 'neuralgia' in the nineteenth century. Both the clinical entity and its theorization varied a good deal. Their main thesis is that when the term was coined it meant intermittent severe pain following the course of a peripheral nerve. Alam & Merskey found that the meaning of the term expanded greatly between 1840 and 1880, so that by the 1870s it could refer to almost any unexplained pain, regardless of distribution, quality or pattern. After 1880 it rapidly resumed a usage close to that of 1802. In my opinion they struggle to account for this expansion and subsequent contraction of meaning. My own view is that Romberg was responsible for expanding the usage and Gowers for restricting it. This will be argued in detail when these primary sources are discussed in Chapters 4 and 6. They also could have made more of the fact that the terms *névralgie* and *névrose* both came to prominence in French medical writings around 1800. While Rey has hinted that pain without lesion was the major challenge to the new clinical method, Alam & Merskey say nothing on this striking chronology.

Before leaving secondary sources on the history of neuralgia it is worth drawing attention to an aside by the historian López Piñero. He asserts that neuralgia was dropped from the category of neurosis between 1850 and 1880.[43] Alam & Merskey's more detailed research places this reclassification at the later date.

## History of Neurosis

López Piñero[44] has written the most scholarly and authoritative account of the conceptual history of neurosis to date. Unfortunately this text is so tightly confined to the history of ideas that all discussion of the technological constraints on theorization, or the professional contexts in which theories were developed, is left out. This must put in question the rather crisp blocks of theory that he has identified. Nonetheless, his book is most valuable for sketching the conceptual landscape and offering some technical terms to characterize various theoretical schools and positions. For example, he coined expressions such as 'the principle of negative lesion', 'speculative functionalism' and 'functional localisation' which I have found a useful shorthand to adopt.

He, like Clarke & Jacyna,[45] identifies three schools of thought in the early nineteenth century: anatomo-clinical, pathophysiological and *naturphilosophie*. His account starts with Pinel's adoption of Cullen's term 'neurosis'. In the late eighteenth century Cullen named disturbances of sense and motion in the absence of fever or topical change of organs 'neuroses'. López Piñero argues that Pinel borrowed the term but, under the influence of Bichat's pathological anatomy, drew particular attention to the absence of a structural lesion in his definition of neurosis. Thus it became a diagnosis of exclusion, based on what the historian calls 'the principle of negative lesion'. For the anatomo-clinicians who followed, neurosis was therefore a class that was sure to shrink gradually away as more and more lesions were identified through the physical examination of patients in life and after death. However, it quickly became apparent that, despite the best efforts of pathological anatomy, many symptoms lacked structural lesions. This fact threatened to undermine the new method. Broussais 'saved' the new paradigm by suggesting that some lesions were invisible and that pathology could be *process* rather than appearance. Thus functional, rather than structural, lesions underlay these problematic Pinelian *névroses*. López Piñero reminds us that Broussais had absolutely no empirical evidence to support his opinion that an invisible pathophysiological process, 'irritation', was everywhere by dubbing this position 'speculative functionalism'.

The next step in the history of neurosis in France was Georget's effort to overthrow the Pinelian concept and to redefine the neuroses by their *positive* clinical features such as chronicity, an intermittent course, a negligible mortality despite the apparent gravity of suffering and so on. López Piñero argues that this redefinition was ignored in Britain and the term and concept of neurosis dropped there around 1850. Later developments included those authors who insisted that the functional lesions in neuroses must be confined to the nervous system ('functional localisers') and Bernard's demonstration of functional lesions with curare in the laboratory in the 1860s. Finally López Piñero mentions Charcot's explanation of hysteria in terms of transient dynamic lesions and his further efforts to identify pathognomonic clinical features such as *belle indifférence* and the 'glove and stocking' distribution of sensory loss.

Turning to histories of individual neurotic syndromes, the striking feature is the mismatch between the quite enormous secondary literature on hysteria and the relative paucity of work on anxiety, phobias, obsessive-compulsive neurosis, hypochondria, spinal irritation, neurasthenia and so on. Micale has reviewed the historiography of hysteria comprehensively[46, 47] and speaks of the 'new hysteria studies'. He has made a number of criticisms of this literature. He deplores the tiresome antagonism between historians and clinicians, the excessive attention to the spectacular manifestations of Charcotian hysteria at the expense of more common, but less dramatic, forms (such as pain) and the neglect of the large nineteenth-century British medical and surgical literature on hysteria. My work attempts to respond to these complaints. The smaller literature on the other neuroses will be mentioned at relevant points in the body of this book.

## History of Neurology as a Clinical Specialty

McHenry,[48] a standard history of neurology, provides some landmarks that are of relevance to us. He identifies Romberg's *Handbook* of 1840–46 as the first textbook of neurology, states that bedside neurological examination was conceived in the period 1870–1900 and that the specialty began with the appointment of Charcot to his chair in 1882. Sensory examination did not become very meaningful until the early 1890s, after detailed studies of patients with syringomyelia and Brown–Séquard syndrome had clarified the crossed afferent tract for pain. Vibration sense and joint position sense were examined at the bedside as indicators of dorsal column integrity from 1903 onwards. He also mentions the limitations of early-nineteenth-century morbid anatomy of the nervous system: for example, infarction and haemorrhage were not distinguished until after 1850. Spillane[49] also gives examples of the rudimentary nature of post mortem examination: brains were preserved in alcohol in the 1800s but microscopy of brain only began in 1838, serial sections in the 1840s and the technique of Wallerian degeneration (for tracing tracts of nerves) was not introduced until the 1850s. These are some of the technological constraints on theory that López Piñero[50] did not include in his discussion of ideas about lesions and neurosis.

Spillane[51] depicts mid-century 'neurology' as an observational, rather than analytic, discipline. He explains how ophthalmoscopy, though invented by Helmholtz in 1850, was introduced to British neurology by Clifford Allbutt after 1871. Testing of tendon reflexes is attributed to Westphal and Erb (around 1875) and Babinski's plantar sign dates from 1896. Keele[52] also portrays bedside neurological examination as a late-nineteenth-century development:

In the examination of the nervous system there was very little progress during the first half of the nineteenth century. In this sphere gross morbid anatomy failed; such changes as were found were incomprehensible...It was largely owing to Charcot that meticulous correlation of symptoms and morbid anatomical changes began to make sense.[53]

To summarize, it seems clear that analytical bedside neurological examination was developed between 1870 and 1903, with techniques for sensory examination appearing last. My reading of case histories provided an opportunity to comment further on the evolution of bedside sensory examination in the nineteenth century.

Turning now to the demarcation between the professions of neurology and psychiatry, Bynum[54] and Reynolds[55] are important sources. Bynum emphasizes international variation in the histories of these specialties. In Germany there was a strong neuropsychiatric tradition at mid-century, epitomized by Griesinger and Meynert, while in Britain 'a formal psychiatric profession developed in the first half of the nineteenth century, decades before medical specialties such as ...neurology.' By the 1880s there was 'a structurally oriented neurology that had gradually left the care of the nervous patient to ...gynaecologists, general physicians and office-based psychiatrists.' Reynolds[56] concurs:

by the end of the century neurological textbooks were firmly rooted in the new anatomy and pathology and to a much smaller extent on physiological principles, that is, on structure more than function.

He claims that the conventional nineteenth-century meaning of the term 'functional' was 'absence of or undetected brain pathology'. Hughlings Jackson proposed a more active referent for the term: loss of function or overfunction due to destructive or discharging lesions. The words 'functional' and 'neurosis' were shortly 'hijacked' by post-Freudian psychiatry. Reynolds then bemoans the subsequent failure of nosologists to maintain valuable distinctions between motor, sensory, psycho- and reflex neuroses.

Thus a 'nervous patient' might have been under the care of a doctor from either specialty at different points in the century, and this might vary across national contexts. This important consideration necessitates the selection of primary sources from a range of specialties. In the case of lesionless pain, the professional context in which patients were seen was wider still. As Merskey & Spear[57] and Micale[58] have rightly emphasized, surgeons and physicians cared for them in the first half of the century in Britain. Goldstein[59] has described the 'turf war' in France between physicians and alienists over the care of hysterics in the same period.

## History of Experimental Psychology

Boring[60] takes an interesting position with respect to the German concept of *Gemeingefühl* and von Frey's importance in the history of pain. We have seen that both Keele[61] and Rey[62] portrayed von Frey as a 'villain' who was responsible for the oversimplified, reductionist view of pain as a sensation running along a rigid anatomical pathway. In addition, Keele pointed to German overstimulation theories, premised on the concept of bodily sensation, as an important parallel tradition to the elucidation of specific pain pathways. Boring, in diametric opposition to these views, speaks of Weber, Erb, Blix and Goldscheider all clinging to an unhelpful idea, that pain was one aspect of a catch-all notion of *Gemeingefühl* or common sensibility, that impeded scientific progress. Von Frey's identification of 'pain spots' as free nerve endings in 1894, and his insistence that pain is a sensory modality in its own right, is depicted by Boring as liberating pain research from the murky concepts of German Romanticism.

## Conclusions

The secondary literature points to a large number of primary sources relevant to our topic and to the need to include medical writings from a wide range of professional contexts: British surgeons and physicians from the early decades of the century, French alienists of the middle decades, German Romantic psychiatrists and physiologists, neurologists, psychiatrists and early psychoanalytic authors.

A number of arguments demand further consideration. Foremost among these is the widely-held view[63-65] that the rise of a reductionist neurophysiology led to loss of appreciation of the psychological dimensions of pain and to lesionless pain being dismissed as imaginary. We have seen that there was a parallel tradition, grounded in German Romanticism, in which pain was considered as a bodily sensation, an aspect of common sensibility, rather than as a sensory modality in its own right. This complicates the 'rise of neuroscience' argument and directs us to a re-examination of the seminal work of Johannes Müller and E.H.Weber. One extension of the argument, that interest in lesionless pain was at an all time low by the end of the century, strikes me as particularly weak. That position can only be sustained by systematically ignoring research into the neuroses in the 1890s, including the beginnings of psychoanalytic thought.

The other important general argument is Shorter's claim that somatized motor symptoms were common at the mid-century, while sensory symptoms, such as lesionless pain, came to the fore later.[66] This will be challenged and a case made for the sustained presence of a rather historically invariant clinical syndrome of chronic pain without lesion.

Finally this review reveals the scope for contributing to the history of bedside sensory examination in the nineteenth century and some comments on this theme will be included when case histories are presented.

The secondary literature draws attention to a number of historiographical pitfalls: anachronism, retrospective diagnosis, overgeneralizing from a small case history base, overstating historical variance and social constructionism, failing to attend to the professional context in which theory was written and to the technological constraints that shaped such theory and saying far too much about Charcot and Freud, at the expense of other equally influential authors. My methodological response to these warnings will now be briefly described.

### Methodological Remarks

Formidable difficulties surround any attempt to write a history of pain without lesion. The research strategy must be situated with respect to methodological polarities common to all contemporary history of medicine, such as diachronic versus synchronic and 'internal' versus 'external' accounts. Micale[67, 68] and Berrios[69, 70] have offered spirited defences of diachronic intellectual history of psychiatry as well as prescribing some historiographic guidelines for such work. It is important to make distinctions between the history of words (historical semantics), concepts (conceptual history) and clinical objects (behavioural palaeontology).[71] The method I have adopted strives to encompass all three.

I begin by arguing for the appearance of an important and enduring problem around 1800, namely the conundrum of pain without structural lesion. In Chapter One I argue in detail that the problem was a product of the emergence of a new clinical method in which physical signs in vivo and structural pathology post mortem were considered of greater value than symptoms. The next step is to assume, as a research strategy, that the problem continued to provoke theoretical innovation throughout the nineteenth century. Once this historically invariant problem is accepted as a given, diachronic review of the theories put up to explain it (conceptual history) and of the terms used to name it (historical semantics) becomes possible. Perhaps more intriguingly, this methodology renders the historical stability of the clinical phenomenon of lesionless pain (the behavioural palaeontology) an open question to be answered by textual research using case histories.

I have shied away from writing a history of 'psychogenic pain' because this would be ahistorical. The term was not coined until 1904, and singling out nineteenth-century 'anticipations' of the concept would relegate the research to a further contribution to the well-trodden and unsatisfactory genre of 'prehistories of psychoanalysis'. A history of Pain Disorder (as defined in DSM IV)[72] would also be anachronistic since this syndrome includes diagnostic criteria, such as exclusion of a primary mood disorder and the need for evidence of psychological conflict, that reflect rather recent ideas.

Micale[73] has emphasized that the choice of primary sources is an issue of paramount importance in any diachronic intellectual history. The method of selection of primaries must be described and justified. I identified primary materials that might contain discussion of the problem of pain without lesion in three ways: by organic reference searching of the secondary sources, by computerized search of some of the nineteenth-century medical literature and by hand searching the Catalogue of the Surgeon General of 1889. The computerized search was of the holdings of the Wellcome Institute's library using an in-house software system called 'WILDCAT'. Among the keywords searched over the period 1800–1914 were: pain, chronic pain, hypochondria, hysteria, neurosis, neuralgia, spinal irritation, rheumatism, headache, spine, backache, abdominal pain and dysmenorrhoea. Primaries were selected from just three countries – Britain, France and Germany – because most important contributions to nineteenth-century neurology and psychiatry came from these, and authors throughout Northern Europe were generally aware of each others' work. This is not to argue that these texts are homogeneous, rather that they are similar enough to justify studying them as a group. My research is confined to elite theory and my chosen method does not reveal much about the history of therapeutic practice. I have made an effort to use the numerous case histories as an opportunity to say something about the evolution of diagnostic practice and bedside examination of chronic pain patients.

There is an inevitable tension between the number of texts described and discussed and the depth of 'external' context provided. I have only included enough contextual material to indicate the professional biographies of medical theorists and some of the technological constraints on the answers they devised to the problem of pain without lesion. My work says almost nothing about social, political or institutional history and thus falls short of Micale's ideal of a 'sociosomatic' history of medicine.[74]

## Notes

1   Merskey & Spear, 1967, *Pain: psychological and psychiatric aspects.*
2   Morris, 1991, *The Culture of Pain.*
3   Shorter, 1992, *From Paralysis to Fatigue: a history of psychosomatic illness in the modern era.*
4   Merskey & Spear, 1967, *Pain: psychological and psychiatric aspects.*
5   Merskey, 1979, *The Analysis of Hysteria.*
6   Rey, 1993, 236, *History of Pain.*
7   Morris, 1991, 4, *The Culture of Pain.*
8   *Ibid.*, 112.
9   Foucault, 1973, *The Birth of the Clinic: an archaeology of medical perception.*
10   Jewson, 1976, *The disappearance of the Sick man from medical cosmology, 1770–1870.*
11   Morris, 1991, 104, *The Culture of Pain.*
12   Briquet, 1859, *Traité clinique et thérapeutique de l'hystérie.*
13   Risse, 1988, *Hysteria at the Edinburgh Infirmary: the construction and treatment of a disease, 1770–1800*
14   Merskey & Watson, 1979, *The lateralisation of pain.*
15   Shorter, 1992, *From Paralysis to Fatigue: a history of psychosomatic illness in the modern era.*
16   *Ibid.*, preface.
17   *Ibid.*
18   Romberg, 1853, *A Manual of the Nervous Diseases of Man,* second edition.
19   Shorter, 1992, 26, *From Paralysis to Fatigue.*
20   *Ibid.*, 150–200.
21   Keele, 1957, *Anatomies of Pain.*
22   Rey, 1993, *History of Pain.*
23   Keele, 1957, 110–11, *Anatomies of Pain.*
24   Gowers, 1886, *A Manual of Diseases of the Nervous System* Quoted in Keele, 1957.
25   Keele, 1957, 183, *Anatomies of Pain*
26   Melzack & Wall, 1965, *Pain mechanisms: a new theory.*
27   Merskey & Spear, 1967, *Pain: psychological and psychiatric aspects.*
28   Morris, 1991, *The Culture of Pain.*
29   Rey, 1993, *History of Pain.*

30  *Ibid.*

31  Mullan, 1988, *Sentiment and sociability: the language of feeling in the eighteenth century.*

32  Foucault, 1973, *The Birth of the Clinic.*

33  Bichat, 1801, *Anatomie Générale.* Quoted in Rey, 1993, 111–13.

34  Rey, 1993, 113–15, *A History of Pain.*

35  *Ibid.*, 148.

36  *Ibid.*, 150.

37  Merskey & Spear, 1967, *Pain: psychological and psychiatric aspects.*

38  Morris, 1991, *The Culture of Pain.*

39  Rey, 1993, 245, *History of Pain.*

40  *Ibid.*, 239–41.

41  *Ibid.*, 242.

42  Alam & Merskey, 1994, *What's in a name? The cycle of change in the meaning of neuralgia.*

43  López Piñero, 1983, 72, *Historical Origins of the Concept of Neurosis.*

44  *Ibid.*

45  Clarke & Jacyna, 1987, *Nineteenth-century Origins of Neuroscientific Concepts.*

46  Micale, 1989, *Hysteria and its historiography: a review of past and present writings.*

47  Micale, 1995, *Approaching Hysteria: disease and its interpretations.*

48  McHenry, 1969, *Garrison's History of Neurology.*

49  Spillane, 1981, *The Doctrine of the Nerves: chapters in the history of neurology.*

50  López Piñero, 1983, *Historical Origins of the Concept of Neurosis.*

51  Spillane, 1981, *The Doctrine of the Nerves: chapters in the history of neurology.*

52  Keele, 1963, *The Evolution of Clinical Methods in Medicine.*

53  *Ibid.*, 81–82.

54  Bynum, 1985, *The nervous patient in eighteenth- and nineteenth-century Britain: the psychiatric origins of British neurology.*

55  Reynolds, 1992, *Structure and function in neurology and psychiatry.*

56  *Ibid.*

57  Merskey & Spear, 1967, *Pain: psychological and psychiatric aspects.*

58  Micale, 1989, *Hysteria and its historiography: a review of past and present writings.*

59  Goldstein, 1987, *Console and Classify: the French psychiatric profession in the nineteenth century.*

60  Boring, 1942, *Sensation and Perception in the History of Experimental Psychology.*

61  Keele, 1957, *Anatomies of Pain.*

62  Rey, 1993, *History of Pain.*

63  Merskey & Spear, 1967, *Pain: psychological and psychiatric aspects.*

64  Morris, 1991, *The Culture of Pain.*

65  Rey, 1993, *History of Pain.*

66  Shorter, 1992, *From Paralysis to Fatigue.*

67  Micale, 1990a, *Hysteria and historiography: the future perspective.*

68  Micale, 1995, *Approaching Hysteria: disease and its interpretations*

69  Berrios, 1992, *Research into the history of psychiatry.*

70  Berrios, 1994, *Historiography of mental systems and diseases.*

71  Berrios, 1992, *Research into the history of psychiatry.*

72  DSM-IV, American Psychiatric Association, 1994

73  Micale, 1995, ch. 2, *Approaching Hysteria: disease and its interpretations.*

74  *Ibid.*

# 1

## The Birth of a Problem

### 1. The Eighteenth-century Background:
### Sensibility, Sympathy & Nervous Diseases 1750–1800

Bynum[1] has characterized the second half of the eighteenth century as a period in which the hold of Hippocratic humoralism was being eroded and the importance of the nervous system in health and disease increasingly emphasized. This shift was played out in writings on sensibility and sympathy, some of the most famous of which will be briefly summarized as background to our period of interest.

#### Sensibility

Rey is quite clear that 'sensibility was a physiological concept before it was a psychological or aesthetic one'[2] while Mullan[3] highlights the shared vocabulary and, by implication, the interdependence of the literary and medical fields at mid-century. Much can be made of the fact that the author of *The English Malady* of 1733,[4] George Cheyne, was the physician and friend of Samuel Richardson, the novelist of sentiment. Both wrote of sensibility as a blessing and a curse, a result of progress, a sign of intellect and refinement, yet a feature that could take a person close to insanity. Sensibility was also of new importance as the starting point for epistemology in Locke's empiricism and Condillac's sensualism. But, according to Rey, it was the precise definition and the beginnings of measurement of it that were to prove of greatest heuristic value. The starting point of this endeavour is generally taken to be Albrecht von Haller's 1752 lectures to George II's 'Royal Society' in Göttingen.[5]

Haller defined sensibility as follows:

> I call that a sensible part of the human body, which on being touched transmits the impression of it to the soul; and in brutes, in which the existence of a soul is not so clear, I call those parts sensible, the Irritation of which occasions evident signs of pain and disquiet in the animal.[6]

Thus sensibility was a property of a body part. Some parts, such as bone marrow and tendons, did not possess it. Note that from this famous beginning, pain was taken to be the exemplar of sensibility.

Both Robert Whytt in Edinburgh and the Montpellier Vitalists objected to Haller's definition. Whytt regarded sensibility as a property of the brain and spinal cord rather than peripheral nerves. This was for metaphysical, if not theological, reasons according to French[7] and Brazier.[8] Whytt has been depicted as an Animist, arguing for the intervention of an immaterial soul in physiological processes. He was most reluctant to endow mere peripheral nerves with the 'sentient principle', though he did concede that the spinal cord had it. The latter was a conclusion based on observation of decapitated animals and pithed frogs. The Montpellier Vitalists insisted that the whole body has sensibility by virtue of being alive. They could not accept Haller's view that certain parts lacked it. They were also very aware that the conditions of Haller's vivisections might have affected his findings. For example, the pain of a skin incision might obscure the sensibility of the exposed part.[9]

Cullen's concept of sensibility was similar to that of his Edinburgh forbear, Whytt. He too 'placed' sensibility in the brain and spinal cord rather than peripheral body parts. However, Lawrence[10] has convincingly pointed out an additional crucial influence on Cullen's account of sensation from the Scottish philosopher David Hume. Cullen divided mental events into sensations and ideas. Sensations, like Humean 'Impressions', were states of feeling as opposed to Ideas, which were the faint images of these in thought. Sensations were fully determined states of feeling which presented irresistibly to the subject's consciousness. However, ideas came and went from attention, with or without the subject's volition, as imaginings and memories. Cullen split sensations further according to their origin. They might arise from external events (e.g. the cut of a knife) or by internal events (e.g. the passions or emotions) coming to attention. He mentioned a number of factors involved in determining sensations, freely mixing variables as diverse as the physical condition of the nerves and the subject's level of attentiveness. Painful experience generated fear and aversion and influenced mood. 'Sensation then...was the basis of the whole of Cullen's physiology and epistemology'.[11]

That Cullen derived such a complex theory of perception from Hume may surprise those familiar with empiricist readings of the latter's philosophy. However, the proximity of Humean 'Impressions' to the 'sense data' of logical positivism was probably overstated in early twentieth-century histories of philosophy for polemical reasons.

Across the Channel, Condillac's *Traité des Sensations* of 1754[12] had more direct impact than the thought of Locke or Hume. One of his critical disciples, Pierre-Jean-Georges Cabanis, 'was drawn to the questions Condillac had answered inadequately concerning corporeal influences on sensations'.[13] This Parisian Idéologue physician and philosopher was also much influenced by the Montpellier Vitalists, notably Barthez. His most famous exposition of *Sensibilité* was in the *Rapports* of 1798[14] and his ideas were remarkably similar to Cullen's.

Sensibility, for Cabanis, could be modified by a number of Hippocratic variables, such as climate and regime, as well as by age and temperament. He stressed that impressions arising internally were as important as a source of ideas as impressions from the external world. Among internal impressions he included memories and the products of imagination. Cabanis emphasized the crucial role of attention in sensibility. For example, there could be no pain from a serious injury if no attention was paid and, by the same token, pain could arise from excessive attention to fleeting impressions:

> *Nous savons, avec certitude, que l'attention modifie directement l'état local des organes; puis que, sans elle, les lésions les plus graves ne produisent souvent ni la douleur, ni l'inflammation qui leur sont propres; et qu'au contraire, une observation minutieuse des impressions les plus fugitives peut leur donner un caractère important, ou même occasioner quelque-fois des impressions véritables, sans cause réelle extérieure, ou sans objet qui les détermine.*[15]

He goes on to assert that Mesmer cured patients with chronic pain, *les douleurs habituelles*, by redirecting their attention.

So, for Cabanis, pain could arise and be dispelled through the action of memory, attention or imagination. He favoured a competitive model in which external impressions prevented excessive absorption in misleading internal impressions. When the latter took hold the resulting condition was *Hypochondrie*.

In summary, by the 1790s sensibility was seen by elite medical theorists in Edinburgh, Montpellier and Paris as a most important property of nerves, and especially of the brain and spinal cord. Rather than Condillac's passive statue or a Lockean *tabula rasa*, sensibility was determined by the physical condition of the nerves and the mental world of the subject (including his mood, memories and attentiveness) as well as by the flame of the candle that burned him.

## Sympathy

The doctrine of sympathies had been evoked time and again, from the Hippocratic Corpus onwards, to account for certain empirical findings such as the association of headache and nausea or the involvement of the left kidney when the right was diseased. In the late eighteenth century the term acquired an important new connotation. Goldstein[16] has elaborated how sympathy, synonymous now with empathy, took on a social dimension and became central to the appearance of Liberal politics in the Enlightenment. According to her, Adam Smith defined it in 1759 as 'apprehension of the feelings of others' or 'imagination carrying us beyond our own person'. Our natural sympathy with the pain of others was at the very foundation of the Rights of Man. The term 'moral constitution' acquired both corporeal and political resonances that persist to the present. I shall now briefly describe how two medical authors turned to the topic with particular energy and influence, Robert Whytt and Paul-Joseph Barthez.

French[17] and Brazier[18] have emphasized how Whytt's account of the nervous system in the 1760s was an attempt to solve metaphysical and theological problems.[19] For him, normal sympathy, the functional interaction of distant parts of the body, implied the presence of a sentient and regulatory principle – something akin to the soul. Whytt was opposed to investing the most peripheral structures with experiential or regulatory powers and for this reason he opposed Willis's notion that distant parts might interact via anastomoses of nerves in ganglia or plexuses. In fact, in 1681 Willis had identified a large anatomical structure that might mediate such peripheral interaction. He called it the 'Intercostal' and Winslow renamed it the *Grande Sympathique* in 1732. (It is now known as the sympathetic trunk.) Whytt discounted any idea that its function might be independent of the brain and spinal cord. He believed that because parts interacted in a meaningful way, because sympathy was 'wise', it must be mediated centrally, in the brain and spinal cord. Whytt also distinguished 'General Sympathy', awareness of the whole body and its functioning, from 'Specific Sympathies' between particular organs. Pathological sympathy resulted in the 'Nervous Diseases' – hypochondria and hysteria.

Rey[20] has drawn attention to the importance of Barthez's *Nouveaux Éléments de la science de l'homme* of 1778 as a highly influential text on sympathy from a leading Montpellier Vitalist. My research confirms that Bichat responded to it in detail (see below). Barthez delineated three sorts of sympathetic interaction between two organs: with no discernible anatomical connection between the organs, with the structure or function of the organs resembling each other, or with an anatomical connection between the organs. The third of these particularly interested Barthez and he began to document examples of pain at a distance from a diseased part, noting the direction of pain propagation along nerves. He came to the view that, in many examples of such phenomena, the spinal cord was involved but the brain was not.

Rey concludes her discussion of sympathy in the eighteenth century by depicting it as a bridging medical literature between the metastasis of morbific matter in humoral theory and the neuroscience of the nineteenth century. What is very clear is that, by the closing decades, elite physicians agreed that the nervous system was often behind the clinical phenomenon of action at a distance. Pain at a distance from a diseased part was an important and interesting example of this.

### Nervous Diseases

In eighteenth-century Britain and France the term 'nervous disease' meant hysteria in women and hypochondria in men. This usage continued from Blackmore's *A Treatise of the Spleen and Vapours: or, Hypochondriacal and Hysterical Affections* of 1725 [21] until Cullen rather widened the category of nervous disease and renamed it neurosis in 1769.[22] Mullan[23] and Fischer-Homberger[24] have made some comments on this mid-century literature. Mullan points out that texts before the 1760s were aimed at a rich lay audience, the society physician, generally a sufferer of nerves himself, sharing his experiences with the reader. Whytt and Cullen were the first to write for medical experts. Nervous disease was not madness (unreason), rather it was seen as the all too prevalent price of a highly developed sensibility. The symptoms of hysteria were thought more visible and more transient than those of hypochondria. Fischer-Homberger claims that hypochondria was the 'melancholia' of antiquity, renamed in the light of growing doubt as to the existence of black bile. In fact Blackmore, Cheyne and Whytt all favoured the nervous system as the cause of hypochondria, not the 'hypochondriac organs' (spleen, stomach or liver) Boerhaave had blamed.

I shall précis Lawrence's account of the views of Whytt and Cullen on nervous diseases,[25] because these ideas represent useful background to the Pinelian concept of neurosis that is of great importance in my argument. In the *Observations* of 1764,[26] Whytt divided the causes of acquired nervous disease into proximate and ultimate. The former included a by-now rather standard list of retained evacuations, fatigue, sloth, luxury and morbid matter in the blood. The ultimate cause was dysfunction of the 'Sentient Principle', resulting in pathological sympathies and morbid sensibility. In hypochondria, for example, this would mean low mood, due to the effects of the bowel on the brain, and abdominal pain, due to the effects of prolonged melancholy on intestinal spasm. Later Cullen did away with these proximate causes and pathological sympathies altogether, asserting that dysfunction of the nervous system underlay a wide range of clinical pictures. This position has been dubbed 'neural pathology'. In the nosology of 1769[27] he called the large class of nervous disorders the 'Neuroses'. This class included paralysis, mania, melancholia, dyspepsia, hypochondria and hysteria.

## 2. Bichat and the Birth of Clinicopathological Correlation

According to Bynum,[28] the theories of the Montpellier Vitalists bore fruit in the physiological research of Marie-François-Xavier Bichat. In fact, Bichat's father was a Montpellier-trained surgeon of the Barthez school. After studying surgery with Petit in Lyon, Bichat moved to Paris, arriving at the height of the Terror.[29] He became the favourite pupil of the innovative surgeon Desault at the *Hôtel-Dieu* in the 1790s, where he saw attempts made to correlate pathological findings at autopsy with clinical symptoms in life as part of the hospital routine. One other important influence on him was the 'method of analysis' of the philosopher Condillac (for which see Staum[30]). Bichat used variation in sensibility to noxious stimulation as a tool of analysis as he differentiated one tissue system from another:

> What above all else fixed my attention on the diversity of the pains which are found within each system [i.e.tissue], was the question from a man with tremendous spirit and composure, whose thigh had been amputated by Desault. He asked me why the pain that he felt the moment his skin was cut was completely different from the awful feeling that he experienced when his flesh was sectioned – where the nerves which were scattered here and there were injured by the instrument – and why this differed again from that which took place when his marrow was sectioned.[31]

Once Bichat had distinguished the several tissue systems in this way he began to redescribe diseases in terms of visible, structural tissue lesions. The historian who has made most of this discontinuity in medical thought is Michel Foucault. In *The Birth of the Clinic* [32] he argues that Bichat's work represented 'an essential mutation in medical knowledge'. Through tissue lesion disease was 'welded' to the organism rather than being a grouping of symptoms in a nosological table; a 'grammar of signs' replaced a botany of symptoms. Physical signs of underlying lesions became more significant than the relatively unreliable subjective complaints of the patient. A 'medical gaze' replaced the sympathetic ear of the physician, the visual trumped the aural. The question 'What is the matter with you?' was superseded by 'Where does it hurt?'. Foucault claims that the latter question encapsulated the nub of the new discourse, the new anatomoclinical method. The power relations between doctor and patient changed, the patient's body was the new object of interest while the only value of the suffering human subject's speech was to direct the clinician's gaze to the relevant area of the body.

Foucault's account should not be taken up uncritically. For example, Gelfand[33] has emphasized that the 'birth' was preceded by a gestation in the work of surgeons at the *Hôtel-Dieu* in the last decades of the eighteenth century. But historians generally concur that a programme of correlating clinical symptoms with structural pathology post mortem did begin in Paris around 1800.[34-36] It is my contention that symptoms without structural lesions represented a problem for this new anatomoclinical method and, furthermore, that pain without lesion was the most pressing conceptual challenge. The most pressing because pain, in contrast to symptoms such as fatigue or nausea, had a localizing value and spatial localization was at the core of pathological anatomy.

One consequence of the 'birth' of clinicopathological correlation was a rejection of the mid-eighteenth-century nosological order of 'Painful Illnesses' by Bichat and others. Now that pain was seen as a marker of an underlying lesion, and its distribution seen to have localizing value, the notion of a disease order based on pain symptoms alone, as previously advocated by Boissier de Sauvages, was bound to fall. Pain was now a symptom of disease, not a disease in its own right. It had become a marker of something else – structural lesion. As Rey has pointed out,[37] the rejection of de Sauvages's diagnostic category may have been overhasty since what he had in mind was a group of conditions characterized by prominent pain in the absence of obvious structural derangement of the body, a scenario that continued to be encountered throughout the nineteenth century as we shall see.

### 3. The Problem of Pain Without Lesion
### – Neurosis and Neuralgia

From roughly 1800 onwards the effort to link symptom to physical sign in vivo or to morbid appearance post mortem became central to elite medical practice in France and Britain. Clarke & Jacyna[38] have summarized some of the limitations of this enterprise in the early nineteenth century, especially concerning the nervous system. Punctate lesions had often spread by the time of autopsy, there was no understanding of decussation of nerves, morbid anatomy was in its infancy and technologically imperfect (microscopic examination of brain began in the 1830s), there was probably no detailed bedside neurological examination until the 1870s or later. Most importantly, there were many symptoms without lesion and lesions without symptoms. It can be argued that among these symptoms without lesion, including fatigue, nausea, dizziness and breathlessness, it was pain without lesion that posed the greatest challenge to the new clinical paradigm.

In fact Bichat was well aware that two classes of disorder lay beyond the scope of his new pathological anatomy: some fevers and nervous disorders:

> all the diseases of the nervous system are generally defects in animal sensibility...very few admit of a disturbance in the organic...Thus has pathological anatomy very little to do with nerves...even when pain exists in the very nervous system itself, as in tic douloureux, there is seldom any organic injury...In general, the diseases which derange the functions of animal life are quite of different nature from those which destroy the harmony of organic life.[39]

He was also very interested in a number of variables that intervened in the not-so-simple relationship between pain and tissue lesion. Firstly, he recognized that the passions could regulate the actions of animal life (i.e. sensation and motion) though they were seated in organic life.[40] He saw this influence of passion over sensation as involuntary. It constituted a man's character and lay beyond the scope of education. Secondly, he considered the effect of repetition or habit on pain sensation, claiming that repeated stimulation lost its novelty over time and so became less painful: 'The nature of pleasure and of pain is to destroy themselves, to cease to exist.'[41]

Bichat recognized, named and theorized both pain at a distance from lesion and pain without lesion. The former phenomenon was a sympathy and the latter a neuralgia.

Bichat discussed examples of pain at a distance from lesion in most detail in the section of *General Anatomy*[42] on sympathies. He begins by taking issue with Barthez, the most systematic contemporary author on the subject, and specifically excluding the 'natural connection in functions' from the field of real sympathy. For example, Bichat could not accept that the influence of nerve on brain or muscle be regarded as a sympathy. Three examples of the kinds of clinical phenomena Bichat accounted for by sympathy will suffice. He stated that two nerves of a pair might sympathise so that a sciatic pain in the left leg of a woman would also appear in the right in bad weather. The headache often associated with stomach disorder provided an example of sympathy between nerve and another organ. Finally, the pain in the glans penis when a bladder stone was present provided a third type. All of these sympathetic pains are explained as misperceptions or illusions:

> when a part is sympathetically affected...the part which is the seat of the essential cause of the pain, first acts upon the brain, either by the nerves, or by some means we are unacquainted with, and...it mistakes this sensation, and refers it to a part from which it has not arisen...These aberrations of animal sensibility then exist entirely in the brain. It is an irregularity, a disturbance in perception.[43]

Thus Bichat saw pain at a distance from lesion, referred pain, as an illusion.

As has been mentioned above, Bichat was aware that many disorders of the nervous system were lesionless and beyond the scope of pathological anatomy. Thus it need be no surprise to find this supposed champion of the new clinical method writing about nervous pains without lesion. He did so in discussions of neuralgia in chapters on the nervous systems of animal and organic life in *General Anatomy*,[44] though much of the conceptual groundwork was described in *Physiological Researches upon Life and Death*.[45] While pain was confined to the realm of animal life, it was proposed that organic sensibility of sufficient intensity could undergo a qualitative conversion into animal sensibility. Thus the ganglionic nervous system could give rise to pain. The pain from parts with ganglionic innervation differed in character from that arising from parts innervated by cerebral nerves: the former was 'deeper, to the heart' (for example, uterine pain).

Bichat argued that physicians should make use of Chaussier's new term neuralgia (*névralgie*) in cases of pain without lesion: 'Physicians do not sufficiently attend to this cause of painful sensations, which are sometimes felt to a very considerable extent, without any apparent injury.'[46] Only pain without lesion of a specific character and severity could be accounted for in this manner. The best examples were tic douloureux and sciatica. However, Bichat went on to propose that other pains without lesion might be explained as neuralgias of the ganglionic nervous system:

> We are aware that there are such things existing as colics, which are essentially nervous, and which undoubtedly are quite independent of all local affections of the serous, mucous and muscular systems of the intestines. These colics are evidently seated in the nerves of the semi-lunar ganglions...; they constitute real neuralgias in the nervous system of organic life: then, these have positively no connection with tic douloureux, sciatica, and the other neuralgias of animal life. The symptoms, the course, the duration etc everything, in a word, is perfectly distinct in both these affections.[47]

It is thus clear that Bichat explained a number of pains without tissue lesion in terms of neuralgias of either the animal or organic nervous systems. He also thought that hypochondria was probably related to the ganglionic nervous system though he never developed this idea.

Philippe Pinel's *Nosographie Philosophique* of 1798[48] influenced Bichat. Bichat even went so far as to credit the older physician with inspiring his tissue concept.[49] But Pinel, in turn, was most impressed by Bichat's thought and considered the problem of lesionless symptoms in successive editions of the *Nosographie*. He had translated Cullen's nosology and now borrowed the term neurosis (*névrose*) to name lesionless symptoms. The absence of tissue lesion became central to a new Pinelian concept of neurosis. The Spanish historian López Piñero[50] has dubbed this 'the principle of negative lesion' and contrasted it with Cullen's concept. While Cullen used the term neurosis for disorders of sensation and movement in the absence of fever, Pinel put a novel and special emphasis on the absence of Bichatian structural lesion. In the fifth edition of 1813 it was expressed thus: '4th CLASS: *NÉVROSES: Lésions du sentiment et du mouvement, sans inflammation ni lésion de structure*'.

In the first edition of 1798, neuroses characterized by pain were classified across two orders of the class: hypochondria, hysteria and melancholia were *Vesanies non fébriles* while various painful conditions were *Anomalies locales des fonctions nerveuses*. This latter order included *cardialgie, angine de la poitrine, colique du Poitou* and *affections arthritiques*. Such a classification was close to Cullen's. But by the fifth edition the neuroses were more explicitly discussed as lesionless symptoms and neuralgias included. Painful conditions were split across three of the five orders now: *des fonctions cérébrales* (including hypochondria), *de la locomotion* (including neuralgias) and *des fonctions nutritives* (including colics and cardialgia).

What I want to emphasize from this material is the simultaneous appearance of two new terms in Paris around 1800. Pinel borrowed the word *névrose* in 1798 and Chaussier coined the term *névralgie* in 1801. Thus the problem of lesionless symptoms, and in particular lesionless pain, both arose and was named with the birth of anatomoclinical method.

### 4. The Pains of Hypochondria in the writings of French Alienists *c.*1820

Merskey & Spear[51] made the important historical observation that it was surgeons and physicians, rather than asylum doctors or alienists, who encountered and described pain without lesion in the early decades of the nineteenth century. This has guided my selection of primary sources. However, Goldstein[52] has described a local turf war that developed in France as alienists, especially Esquirol's pupils, sought to capture the care of neurotics from physicians. Most British and German 'psychiatrists' of this period confined their efforts to the care of the institutionalized insane rather than contemplating the problem of lesionless somatic symptoms. For example, Heinroth, the German 'psychiatrist', specifically excluded diseases of the senses, such as the hallucinations of hysteria and hypochondria, from the category of mental illness on the grounds that there is no permanent loss of reason in these conditions.[53] In France, perhaps because of the special position of Pinel who bridged the medical and 'psychiatric' camps, at least one elite group of alienists in and around Paris wrote about neurosis.

#### Falret

Jean-Pierre Falret trained in the Faculties of Medicine at Montpellier and Paris. He was a student at the *Salpêtrière* around 1815 and became one of a group that Goldstein has dubbed 'Esquirol's Circle'. Together with Voison he founded a *maison de santé* for the insane at Vauves in 1822. In the same year his book *De l'hypochondrie et du suicide* was published[54]. There are two essays but only the second, on hypochondria, will be described here.

Falret wrote the essay to establish, once and for all, that

hypochondria is a disorder of the brain rather than of the stomach or any other abdominal organ. He saw himself as putting flesh on the bones of an idea expressed by Georget, his contemporary, and arguing against the views of previous authors, most notably Louyer-Villermay (who had published on the subject between 1802 and 1816). One of the key arguments Falret uses is the predominance of mental and nervous symptoms over digestive symptoms in hypochondria. To this end, when he described the symptoms of the condition in detail, he began with sensory symptoms and only mentioned disturbances of the digestive, respiratory and circulatory systems much later. He stated that headache (*céphalalgie*) was usually present in hypochondria and, together with insomnia, often the very first symptom. The pain could be frontal, occipital, on the top of the head or all over it.

> *Les malades disent alors qu'ils ont la tête lourde et comme accablée sous le poids d'un fardeau, d'une calotte de plomb; ou...ils se plaignent qu'elle est comprimée lateralement comme dans un étau.*

In addition to head pain *'les malades accusent les douleurs les plus diverses pour leur siége et pour leur nature'* and sometimes report extraordinary sensations such as the movements of a grass-snake or fish inside their body. All these sensory experiences are regarded as hallucinations by Falret, that is *'de phénomènes cérébraux qui ne sont pas provoqués par la lésion des extrémités sentantes'.* He goes on to highlight overpreoccupation with health, apathy, social withdrawal, loss of all capacity for enjoyment, variable mood and self-examination as other important symptoms of hypochondria.

Falret regarded hypochondria as a disorder with an hereditary aspect, an age of onset between 25 and 60 years and affecting men more than women. He offered two explanations for the sex distribution: women are less likely to fatigue their intellect with profound meditation and their more energetic sensibility and passions give rise to the convulsive symptoms of hysteria rather than hypochondria. Causes of hypochondria include mental overwork, strong emotions and masturbation. Those studying the *beaux-arts* are more at risk than those pursuing the exact sciences because the imagination is used more in the former. One exception to this is medical students. Falret gives examples of medical students becoming preoccupied by the possibility of suffering the diseases that they were learning about, including his own concern that he may be suffering tuberculosis after lectures at the Medical Faculty in Montpellier. The emotions that Falret lists as causes of hypochondria include *chagrin, crainte* (fear) and *l'ennui* (boredom). Indirect causes are listed briefly: alcohol abuse, purgative abuse, too much tea or sugar and cold drinks.

Falret cites 12 case histories and comments on each. As a rhetorical device these cases are taken from the work of his adversary, Louyer-Villermay. Pain is mentioned among the symptoms in six cases. Two patients had been medical students and one a pharmacist.

A section of the essay is dedicated to post mortem findings but only two autopsies are reported, one from his own experience and one from Louyer-Villermay. He prefaced these reports with the comment that one would not expect to find lesions in hypochondria as it was a nervous system disorder. Any structural changes in the viscera should be seen as secondary complications of the condition. One of the brain autopsies is sufficiently detailed to give an idea of contemporary practice:

> *La dure mère était pale, et ses sinus presque vides de sang. Une sérosité assez abondante, ayant un aspect gélatineux, existait entre l'arachnoide et a pie-mère; cette dernière membrane était épaissie et adhérait fortement dans plusieurs endroits à la substance cérébrale.*

> *En coupant le cerveau par tranches, le sang suintait de tous les points de sa surface, surtout vers les lobes moyens; quatre onces environ de sérosité jaunâtre furent trouvée dans les ventricules.*

> *La consistence du cerveau était à peu près la même que dans l'état ordinaire; peut-être cependant cet organe était-il un peu plus mon.*

It is interesting to find that the technique of macroscopic serial sectioning of brain was used by the early 1820s since Spillane[55] points out that serial sections were not examined microscopically until the 1840s.

Turning to the treatment of hypochondria, Falret argued for the moral treatment favoured by Pinel. The first and indispensable step was to gain the confidence of the patient. This was best achieved, he suggested, by sympathizing with their pain and listening with interest and attention to the lengthy enumeration of their woes. As time went on the physician modified his language and began to challenge the patient. The aim was to divert the patient from preoccupation with himself through encouraging him to mix socially, find new interests or undertake journeys.

## Georget

Georget was an exact contemporary of Falret and an even more highly favoured student of Esquirol. He enrolled in the Faculty of

Medicine in Paris in 1813 and was at the *Salpêtrière* between 1817 and 1819. He won a prize for an essay on the organic lesions seen in *Folie,* wrote a thesis on the causes of madness and was rewarded with a post at Esquirol's own *maison de santé* in Ivry, near Paris. His *Recherches sur les malades nerveuses en général, et en particulier sur le siége, la nature et le traitement de l'hystérie, de l'hypochondrie, de l'épilepsie et de l'asthme convulsif* of 1821[56] encompasses his thought on four conditions that fell short of outright madness. As Falret said, Georget favoured the brain rather than the viscera as the seat of hypochondria, and to this end suggested it be renamed *cérébropathie.* He listed the symptoms that he saw as indicative of a chronic cerebral disorder: insomnia, headache and hallucinations. Pain figured largely among the latter:

> *Les malades se plaignent presque constamment des sensations douloureuses les plus diverses et les plus variables pour le siége et la nature...Je suis convaincu que la plupart du temps, ces sensations sont de véritables hallucinations, le resultat de l'action morbide du cerveau.*

His evidence for the hallucinatory nature of these pains was first that the painful organ was healthy and second that the organ affected was readily altered by contact with another patient in pain. Georget offered a similar, but shorter, list of causes to Falret and gave no reports of autopsies in hypochondria.

The companion essay in the same volume, *De la physiologie du système nerveux, et spécialement du cerveau,*[57] includes some 10 pages on pain in a section headed *Relations sympathiques du système nerveux.* This passage is of considerable interest as it seems to demonstrate that Georget drew a distinction between the physical pain of diseased tissue and moral pain. He gives a by now orthodox Bichatian account of how physical pain varies according to the type and condition of diseased tissue. He acknowledges that *les dispositions cérébrales* profoundly influence perception of physical pain (for example idiots feel little while women with the vapours feel much). However, he places moral pain to one side of his physiological writing in the same volume as his account of the hallucinatory pains of hypochondria. Georget thus drew a clear distinction between mental and physical pain. Hallucinated pains are physical pains lacking external referents and arising from a diseased brain. The conceptualization of pain without lesion as an hallucination in these writings by Falret and Georget obviously owes everything to their master, Esquirol's, relatively recent and highly influential 'invention' of the concept of hallucination as percept without object.

## Summary

The eighteenth-century concepts of sensibility and sympathy have been briefly sketched. I have then argued that the birth of anatomoclinical medicine in Paris around 1800, in part a product of Bichat's physiological research on pain sensibility, rendered symptoms lacking structural tissue lesions sharply problematic. Pain without lesion was the most pressing challenge facing the new programme of clinicopathological correlation since pain was supposed to have value as a localizing symptom. New terms and concepts, notably a new definition of neurosis and the coining of the term neuralgia, were invoked to explain this phenomenon. Older terms and concepts, such as sympathy and hypochondria, were modified in the light of it. Finally I have presented a brief exposition of early French 'psychiatric' interest in neurosis. Esquirol's pupils regarded the pains of hypochondria as hallucinations, the product of a diseased brain.

## Notes

1. Bynum, 1994, *Science and the Practice of Medicine in the Nineteenth Century.*
2. Rey, 1993, 102, *History of Pain.*
3. Mullan, 1988, *Sentiment and Sociability: the language of feeling in the eighteenth century.*
4. Cheyne, 1733, *The English Malady; or a treatise of nervous diseases of all kinds.*
5. Brazier, 1984, 118, *A history of Neurophysiology in the 17th and 18th centuries.*
6. *Haller, 1753. Cited in Brazier, 1984.*
7. French, 1969, ch 4, *Robert Whytt, the Soul and Medicine.*
8. Brazier, 1984, 133, *A History of Neurophysiology in the 17th and 18th centuries.*
9. Rey, 1993, 126–8, *History of Pain.*
10. Lawrence, 1984, 323–3, *Medicine as culture: Edinburgh and the Scottish enlightenment.*
11. *Ibid.*, 330.
12. Condillac, 1754, *Traité des sensations.*
13. Staum, 1980, *Cabanis: enlightenment and medical philosophy in the French Revolution.*
14. Cabanis, 1798, *Rapports du physique et du moral de l'homme.*
15. Cabanis, 1815, 117-8, *Rapports,* 3rd edition.
16. Goldstein, 1993, *Empathy as a category in the historiography of*

*psychiatry.*

17. French, 1969, *Robert Whytt, the Soul and Medicine.*

18. Brazier, 1984, *A History of Neurophysiology in the 17th and 18th centuries,*

19. Whytt, 1764, *Observations on the nature, causes and cure of those diseases which are commonly called nervous, hypochondriac or hysteric.*

20. P.-J. Barthez, 1778, *Nouveaux éléments de la science de l'homme.* Quoted in Rey, 1993, 138–40.

21. Blackmore, 1725, *A treatise of the spleen and vapours: or, hypochondriacal and hysterical affections.*

22. Cullen, 1769, *Synopsis nosologiae methodicae.*

23. Mullan, 1988, ch 5, *Sentiment and Sociability: the language of feeling in the eighteenth century.*

24. Fischer-Homberger, 1972, *Hypochondriasis of the eighteenth century – neurosis of the present century.*

25. Lawrence, 1984, 151–5 & 323–3, *Medicine as culture: Edinburgh and the Scottish Enlightenment.*

26. Whytt, 1764, *Observations on the nature, causes and cure of those diseases which are commonly called nervous, hypochondriac or hysteric.*

27. Cullen, 1769, *Synopsis nosologie methodicae.*

28. Bynum, 1994, 7, *Science and the Practice of Medicine in the Nineteenth Century.*

29. Haigh, 1984, *Xavier Bichat and the medical theory of the eighteenth century.*

30. Staum, 1980, *Cabanis: enlightenment and medical philosophy in the French Revolution.*

31. Bichat, 1824, 164, *General Anatomy, applied to physiology and the practice of medicine*

32. Foucault, 1973, xviii–xix, *The Birth of the Clinic.*

33. Gelfand, 1981, *Gestation of the clinic.*

34. Maulitz, 1987, *Morbid Appearances: the anatomy of pathology in the early nineteenth century.*

35. López Piñero, 1983, *Historical Origins of the Concept of Neurosis.*

36. Clarke & Jacyna, 1987, *Nineteenth-century Origins of Neuroscientific Concepts.*

37. Rey, 1993, 109, *History of Pain.*

38. Clarke & Jacyna, 1987, 22–26, *Nineteenth-century Origins of Neuroscientific Concepts.*

39. Bichat, 1824, page lxxiv, *General Anatomy, applied to physiology and the Practice of medicine.*

40. Bichat, 1809, 52, *Physiological Researches upon life and death.*

41. *Ibid.,* 37.

42. Bichat, 1824, *General Anatomy, applied to physiology and the practice of medicine.*
43. *Ibid.*, 208.
44. *Ibid.*
45. Bichat, 1809, *Physiological Researches upon life and death.*
46. Bichat, 1824, 183, *General Anatomy.*
47. *Ibid., 258.*
48. Pinel, 1798, *Nosographie Philosophique.*
49. Bynum, 1994, 32, *Science and the Practice of Medicine in the Nineteenth Century.*
50. López Piñero, 1983, *Historical Origins of the Concept of Neurosis.*
51. Merskey & Spear, 1967, 6, *Pain: psychological and psychiatric aspects.*
52. Goldstein, 1987, *Console and Classify: the French psychiatric profession in the nineteenth century.*
53. Heinroth, 1818, 24 (1975 translation), *Textbook of disturbances of mental life.*
54. Falret, 1822, *De l'hypochondrie et du suicide.*
55. Spillane, 1981, *The Doctrine of the Nerves: chapters in the history of neurology.*
56. Georget, 1821, *Recherches sur les malades nerveuses en général, et en particulier sur le siége, la nature et le traitement de l'hystérie, de l'hypochondrie, de l'épilepsie et de l'asthme convulsif.*
57. Georget, 1821, *De la physiologie du systeme nerveux, et spécialement du cerveau.*

# 2

## A Local Irritation

### Pain Without Lesion in the writings of French and British Physicians and Surgeons: 1820 – 1840

Two lines of elite medical thought stand out as of particular importance for the problem of lesionless pain in the 1820s: Broussais's *médecine physiologique* and the discovery of the Bell–Magendie 'law'. Broussais's speculative physiological writings introduced a temporal dimension to the concept of lesion. Henceforth, structural lesions were seen to be the visible end-stage of an invisible functional process, irritation. This great expansion of the concept of tissue lesion offered one explanation for pains lacking structural lesions and Foucault has gone so far as to claim that it saved the flawed anatomoclinical model in its infancy.[1] I shall go on to suggest that Bell's arguments from anatomy about the role of ganglia, and his interest in facial pain, led him to discriminate the functions of the anterior and posterior spinal nerve roots. By the 1830s, Bell was rewriting traditional sympathies, for example between gut and head, in terms of growing neuroanatomical knowledge and speculative neurophysiology. Bell and Magendies' work on the spinal nerve roots drew the attention of clinicians to 'the spine' as a spatial locus of prime importance in pain patients. The British literature of 1825–40 on 'spinal irritation' will be surveyed to show how the thought of Broussais and Bell was taken up in less well-known monographs.

Next, the lives and work of two British surgeons – Benjamin Brodie and Joseph Swan – will be compared, focusing on their response to the problem of pain without lesion. We shall see how Brodie distinguished neuralgic pain from hysterical pain, of local and constitutional origin respectively, while Swan rejected constitutional causes for local pains. Swan sought trivial lesions at any distance from a pain rather than allow a constitutional explanation. His more 'hardline' application of pathological anatomy is accounted for by his professional biography. The tussle between pragmatic physician–surgeons and anatomical purists over 'surgical hysteria' was still running 30 years later, as a brief glance at the work of Skey and Hilton confirms.

## 1. Broussais on Irritation, Pain and the Passions

François-Joseph-Victor Broussais was, and remains, a controversial figure in medical history. He worked as a naval surgeon in the 1790s before spending five years in Paris as a student of Bichat and Pinel between 1798 and 1803. This culminated in a doctoral thesis on 'hectic fevers'. After a further five years of army doctoring he produced a large *History of the Phlegmasias or Chronic Inflammations* in 1808. This was the first in 'a series of polemical works that rent apart the medical world of post-Napoleonic Paris'.[2] López Piñero has summarized Broussais's approach, which emphasized the continuity between the normal and the pathological and favoured pathophysiological process over morbid anatomical appearance, with the term 'speculative functionalism'. The key concept he developed was 'irritation' as a disorder of function that may or may not develop into a visible inflammatory lesion. The later books in the series included *Examen de la Doctrine generalement admise* (1816), A treatise on physiology applied to pathology (1820) and *De l'irritation et de la folie* (1828). In 1822 he founded a journal called *Annales de la médecine physiologique* and from a base at the Val-de Grâce in Paris from 1814 onwards it is probably fair to describe him as the influential leader of a school of thought: *médecine physiologique*. Towards the end of his career his ideas were increasingly discredited and he became interested in phrenology.

Broussais's thought is of particular importance for the topic of pain without lesion for several reasons. Firstly because he concentrated on fevers and chronic painful conditions: disorders that were most difficult to explain in terms of the new anatomoclinical method. His introduction of 'irritation', a functional as opposed to structural lesion, can be seen as saving the Bichatian programme of clinicopathological correlation by widening the concept of lesion.[3] Secondly because he had a great deal to say about pain. And thirdly because his monolithic reduction of almost all diseases to gastric irritation, for which he was widely criticized in his own day and which has deterred some historians from making a close examination of his writings, can be read as an attempt to place interactions between tissues, passions, percepts and ideas at the centre of pathological processes.

I shall be arguing that Broussais was addressing the clinical observation that pain (and fever) usually precedes the appearance of clinical signs in disease. This fact was of the utmost inconvenience for Bichat's correlative programme. Broussais, far from confining himself to theoretical speculation, gained extensive clinical experience of chronic inflammatory disorders in the years 1803 to 1808. He would have been only too aware of the absence of signs in vivo (or lesions post mortem) to explain symptoms of pain (and fever) in the early stages of these diseases. The concept of irritation was an effort to make sense of this. Furthermore, I shall argue that Broussais extended Bichat's appreciation of the importance of considering the condition of the tissues, as well as the stimuli acting upon them, in interpreting sensation. He extended it to include an assessment of the condition of the whole organism receiving the stimulus, including its emotional state. I have confined myself to a close reading of the 1826 translation of *A Treatise on physiology applied to pathology* since this includes passages defining 'irritation' in detail and a good deal of material on pain and the passions.

Broussais asserted that external bodies acted on tissues causing an increase in the 'organic movements of contractility'. This was 'spasm'. If the spasm attracted fluids to the tissue a 'vital erection' resulted. Vital erections of sufficient intensity constituted Irritation. Irritation was highly mobile, being transmitted from one part of the body to another via the nervous system. The end stage of the process of irritation was inflammation and a detectable lesion.[5]

Broussais then argued that the Bichatian divisions of animal and organic life are inseparable and that the internal state of the viscera (mediated by the ganglionic nervous system) determines the response of an organism to an external stimulus (mediated by the nervous system of animal life). Broussais believed that pain perception was always modified by this:

> pain (of cutting, burning, twisting, distension of skin) is conveyed to the centre of relation which... reflects it back to the viscera; and the brain acts in virtue of the secondary sensations it perceives in them... When the digestive organs are in a healthy condition, the pain occasioned in another part of the body, by the mechanical causes we have already enumerated, may be borne with great fortitude... but if the stomach be affected with inflammation, the pain is felt much more acutely.[6]

Turning to the relationship between sensations and passions, Broussais asserted that 'all our sensations are reducible, for the physiologist, to pleasure or pain'[7] and that all passions are founded on sensations. Broussais explored the apparent distinction between moral and physical pains but concluded that both fell squarely within the province of physiology:

> The physical causes give rise to what are called physical pleasures and pains; whilst moral causes occasion moral pleasures and moral pains. The latter series are felt by the same organs as the pleasures and pains produced by physical causes; consequently, for the physiologist, these pleasures and pains are all physical, since he can only perceive in them a modification of the living tissues. Wherefore, then, do we admit...moral pains? Because we have regard to the agent by which they are produced...by moral pains we understand a state of...uneasiness, perceived in the viscera by the centre of relation, during the exercise of thought...a modification which is nothing more than a state of irritation. But...the physical [stimuli] excite in our organs a state of irritation, similar to that produced in them by moral causes, and thus give rise to the perception of physical pains, analogous to like sensations produced by moral causes.[8]

Thus he insists that all pain, however caused, is the perception of visceral irritation. Moreover, it is this visceral dimension, which puts pain in close relation with the passions, that separates the experience of pain in humans from the mere physical pain seen in animals.[9]

Finally, Broussais devoted some 50 pages to detailing the reciprocal relations between pain and the passions. He lists sadness, anger and fear as passions founded on pain and the pains of hypochondria and hysteria as arising from passions. Let us take sadness as an example of the former:

> Sadness is nourished by two sets of causes; first, melancholy thoughts; secondly, a painful sensation in the viscera, and principally in the nerves of the epigastric region[10]... The visceral pains which concur in keeping up sadness, tend likewise to produce dejection of spirits, discouragement, and even despair.[11]

He goes on to remind the reader that anger and fear are fortunately available as alternatives to suicide. In a chapter entitled 'Of the manner in which the exercise of the intellect, the affective movements, and the passions, become causes of disease' the reverse relationship is described. Melancholy, terror, humiliation and anger are all seen as capable of producing painful internal sensation. This may be confined to a 'purely nervous' visceral pain, but more often, and especially if the passion acts chronically, there is actual

> disorganization of the principal viscera... It is in this way, that we

daily see developed and kept up, chronic hypochondriacal gastrites...
Women, whose generative apparatus is very nervous, will experience,
under the influence of similar causes, the symptoms of hysteria[12]... all
individuals who have long been tormented by the mixed passions,
become hypochondriacal or neuropathic. This exaggerated nervous
susceptibility occasions a great deal of obscurity in the diagnosis of
diseases, so that, amid the complaints, terrors, and sufferings of these
unfortunate beings, it is very difficult to ascertain the degree of
alteration existing in their principal organs.[13]

To summarize, Broussais recognized that inflammation was a
dynamic process rather than a static appearance and so was able to
explain the absence of physical signs to account for pain and fever in
the early stages of many chronic diseases. He widened the concept of
lesion to include functional as well as structural disturbance of the
tissues. His preoccupation with visceral irritation can be read as an
extension of Bichat's effort to draw attention to the condition of the
*percipiens* as well as the *perceptum* in the analysis of sensation.
Broussais saw the emotional element of pain perception as
specifically human and described the reciprocal relations between
pain and the passions in detail. It remains to be seen how influential
Broussais's writings were in France and Britain.

### 2. Fourcade-Prunet – *La Médecine Physiologique* applied to Nervous Disorders.

Jean Guillaume Fourcade-Prunet was taught by Broussais and was an
enthusiastic proponent of the new physiological medicine. Writing
from a position in the Faculty of Medicine in Paris in 1826 he set
about applying Broussais's ideas to a range of conditions regarded as
'nervous' in a monograph entitled *Malades Nerveuses des auteurs
reportées a l'irritation de l'encéphale des nerfs cérébro-rachidiens et
splanchniques avec ou sans inflammation.*[14] Fourcade-Prunet sought to
demonstrate the value of the new concept of irritation in accounting
for various nervous disorders, including neuralgia, headache,
hypochondria, asthma, hysteria, satyrism and nymphomania. To put
a gloss on this, he drew attention to the usefulness of functional
lesion in comprehending the neuroses.

He defined neuralgias as idiopathic irritations of the trunks and
branches of cerebrospinal nerves. He pointed out that this failed to
explain the intermittent, paroxysmal pattern of neuralgic pain unless
the disease process was an 'intermittent phlegmasia'. Headache had
two sets of causes: idiopathic [i.e. in the part itself] and sympathetic

[i.e. at a distance]. The former included bright light, noise and prolonged intellectual work acting directly on the head. The latter included gastritis or gastroenteritis acting to cause a 'vital erection' and minor irritation of the encephalon.[15] Chronic gastric irritation could render the brain neuropathic, a state in which sensation and imagination are perverted in the absence of disturbance of rationality. These patients hallucinate, overattend to their bodies and health and tend to use exaggerated descriptive language. They are one and the same as the hypochondriacs of Louyer-Villermay, who is excused for writing in an era before Broussais had drawn attention to the critical role of gastric irritation. Autopsies of such patients often reveal the lesions of chronic inflammation in the abdominal organs. Thus we find Fourcade-Prunet using Broussais's ideas to bridge the opinions of Louyer-Villermay and Georget regarding the seat of hypochondria. In this view both abdominal organs and brain are disturbed. The mental symptoms and the autopsy findings in the abdomen were thus rendered compatible.

### 3. The Bell–Magendie Controversy

Some of the strongest claims for an historical discontinuity in thought about pain focus on Bell and Magendie's work on the spinal roots. For example, Merskey & Spear[16] argue that Bell's work stands at the beginning of a period in which 'findings of neurophysiology' came to predominate over 'psychological insights' in pain theory. Their argument hinges on the view that the identification of an anatomical structure concerned exclusively with sensation, namely the posterior roots of the spinal nerves, was the beginning of a sustained effort to map pain pathways in the body. This reductive enterprise meant that pain became either 'real' (i.e. 'in' anatomical structures) or else 'imaginary'. Merskey & Spear and Morris[17] depict pain research since the 1950s as a rediscovery of psychological insights lost in the course of the nineteenth century. I shall be putting this argument into question throughout this book. One place to start is with Bell's personal and intellectual biography.

Charles Bell was born and educated in Edinburgh, becoming a Fellow of the Royal College of Surgeons of Edinburgh in 1799. Five years later he moved to London to develop his career. His first book, *Essays on the anatomy of expression* of 1806,[18] was a great success and went through many editions. This work is relevant to our purpose for at least three reasons. First, because the logic of this detailed study of facial expression in man and animals in various mental states is similar to the logic Bell used later in his consideration of the functional significance of the ganglia and nerve roots – to glimpse or touch the brain and its workings through a detailed knowledge of anatomy – to move from structure to function. Such argument from anatomy rested on belief in a designed universe (Natural Theology), to which Bynum has drawn attention in the context of early nineteenth-century neurophysiology.[19] Second, the *Essays* are important because while Bell separated bodily pain from the accompanying 'agony of mind' and emotions in some passages, it seems unlikely that he would later reduce human pain experience to a mechanism in a nerve. In fact he seems to value the emotional response to pain in man as the element that separates human pain from that of beasts. Consider these short extracts on pain:

> In man, the action of the frontal muscle and Corrugator Supercilii, and of the orbicular muscle of the mouth, bestows a greater latitude of expression [than animals have]: and if in addition to the action of these muscles, instead of the wide drawn lips, and exposure of the teeth, as in the rage or bodily pain of animals, the mouth is half closed; the lips inflated by the action of the circular fibres, and drawn down by the action of the peculiarly human muscle, the depressor anguli oris, there is then more of agony of mind than of mere bodily suffering; a combination of muscular actions of which animals are incapable.[20] ...The mingling of despair and rage and bodily pain is a very difficult study for the painter.[21]

Thirdly, this book reveals how heavily influenced Bell was by the writings of Bichat as early as 1805. He certainly followed Bichat's division of the nervous system into animal and vital functions.[22] It was this influence that led to his detailed consideration of the anatomy and likely function of ganglia.

Bell lectured on anatomy and surgery at his London home, at Great Windmill Street, at the new Middlesex Hospital and at the College of Physicians. In 1811, before joining the first of these institutions, he privately published a short book entitled *Idea of a New Anatomy of the Brain*,[23] which he distributed among friends. Cranefield[24] and Rice[25] have described the ideas therein and the manner in which they lay largely unnoticed until Magendie's experiments of 1822. The main thrust of Bell's book was to argue that the cerebrum and cerebellum served different functions, the former being involved in Bichat's animal life (sensation and motion), the latter in vital life. In an effort to 'touch' these parts of the brain indirectly and demonstrate their functions, Bell touched the anterior and posterior spinal nerve roots of stunned rabbits. The former caused limb movement, the latter caused no reaction. Bell concluded that his *Idea* was thus confirmed. Magendie, by being less resistant to vivisection in alert animals, interpreted root-sectioning experiments on puppies as proving that anterior roots were concerned with motor function, posterior roots with sensation (see Rey[26] for a comparison of the methods of Bell with Magendie).

In a series of lectures to the Royal Society between 1821 and 1829 the priority dispute with Magendie coloured Bell's presentations to such an extent that the published version, *The Nervous System of the Human Body*, is a minefield for the unwary. Rather than using this text as a source for addressing the priority dispute I shall concentrate on two aspects of it: the discussion of the functional significance of ganglia and the case histories of patients with pain, to be found in the third edition of 1836.[27]

It quickly becomes apparent to the reader that Bell was preoccupied with arguing from anatomy about the function of ganglia and that this, rather than any physiological experimentation, led him to regard the spinal roots as 'double nerves' with differing functions. Many authors of the early nineteenth century saw the ganglia as structures like knots that blocked off the vital functions from awareness and the exercise of will. This view was based on consideration of the ganglionic nervous system. Bell recognized that the cerebro-spinal nerves had ganglia too: '31 pairs of large ganglions, in regular order, and carefully protected...'[28] Bell compared and contrasted the anatomy and function of the fifth and seventh cranial nerves. The former was ganglionated and largely sensory in function (though Bell later discovered a small motor component consistent with its double root), while the seventh nerve was unganglionated and division caused extensive facial paralysis (latterly known as Bell's palsy). He argued from anatomy that ganglionated nerve roots were concerned with sensation and that ganglia were anatomical markers of sensory function rather than blockers of sensation. It is tempting to suggest that an interest in tic douloureux – a pain without lesion – in the early decades of the century, and observation of the effects of surgical divisions of facial nerves, contributed more to Bell's thought than physiological experiment. This view is supported by the case histories that Bell collates in the third edition. It is clear that he had a special interest in facial pain. He was strongly opposed to division of nerve, and especially to amputation, as a treatment in cases of pain as an isolated symptom. What is surprising and striking in some of these case histories is the use Bell makes of 'visceral irritation' to explain pain without lesion. This implies that he was influenced in the early 1830s by Broussais, as he had been by Bichat some 25 years earlier:

> [the ganglionic nervous system] must have powerful, though secret, influences... Are we to admit or to deny this influence of...visceral irritation – in producing external pains?... No man who attends to disease can deny the existence of this influence... the line of connexion is clearly laid down in the anatomy.[29]
> so convinced am I that it is the more direct connexion established betwixt the sympathetic nerve and the fifth that produces this [facial] pain, that I could wish to divide the sympathetic in the neck, if I thought it could be done with safety, which it cannot.[30]

The anatomical relation between the fifth and the sympathetic nerves means 'external pains become significant of internal disease, or more commonly of irritation and disordered function' hence 'the frequent and intimate dependence of a painful affection of the face upon the state of the digestive organs'.

The collection of cases gathered under the heading 'Pains of the nature of tic douloureux in other parts of the frame' offer a further glimpse at Bell's clinical approach to pain without lesion. It was largely unaffected by his famous discovery as this selection illustrate:

Example 1[31]: A lady with a 7 year history of pain in the ankle – 'married on crutches'. No visible indication of disease.

Example 2[32]: Miss D a lady of cultivated mind. She described her suffering in very animated language. She had been confined to her room for years, and passed most of her time kneeling by the bedside. She took in the course of the twenty-four hours five hundred drops of laudanum... I expected to find the hip and thigh one extended ulceration. There was no disease, not the slightest discoloration! However, if we cannot relieve these pains, it is cruelty and ignorance to call them imaginary.

Example 3[33]: A young lady admitted to the Middlesex Hospital the day Bell left that institution. Pain from knee to heel. No disease. A series of amputations of the limb were performed against Bell's written advice, culminating in amputation at the hip. No relief.

Example 4[34]: Pain of right upper limb and breast. 'She acknowledges great depression of spirits'. There was no breast disease. Bell argued that this pain arises 'from a source internal'.

Example 5[35]: A middle-aged gentleman who complains of an excruciating pain seated in the whole back for 4 years. Relieved by firm pressure and walking, exacerbated by the slightest touch. Most doctors assumed the pain 'arose from inflammation of the spinal marrow' and offered local applications. Bell did not agree.

> Such cases are important, when we find so many patients, particularly young ladies, laid for months in the horizontal posture, on account of morbid sensibility in the spine or back.

These cases show Bell's dissatisfaction with dismissing chronic pain without lesion as imaginary and his equal reluctance to invoke the relatively new notion of spinal irritation, which, as I argue below, developed precisely because of the attention now paid to the spinal column in the wake of his famous discovery. Bell seems to have been alert to the possibility that internal causes as diverse as visceral irritation and depression of spirits may be at play in the production of chronic pain.

I hope these few comments on Bell's writings are sufficient to oppose any characterization of him as the first in a line of experimental neurophysiologists who transformed the status of pain so as to dismiss pain without lesion as imaginary. Bell never wrote at length about lesionless pain, except facial pain, but the man he displaced as lecturer at Great Windmill Street in 1812, Benjamin Brodie, did. Before turning to Brodie's *Lectures* of 1837, I shall explore a number of works by less well known British authors who combined aspects of the thought of Bell and Broussais in their accounts of 'spinal irritation'.

### 4. Spinal Irritation 1825–1840

Spinal irritation has been tackled briefly by López Piñero[36] and rather more fully by Shorter[37]. I have re-examined the primary sources used by these historians with particular reference to pain. My argument is that many of these authors made very different use of the thought of Bell, Magendie and Broussais than we do now. It will be proposed that, for them, Bell's work determined the spinal localization of irritation simply by attracting clinicians' attention to 'the spine', and that the full potential of incorporating a temporal dimension into pathology was not realized by these British authors. They were more taken with the explanatory utility of irritation as an invisible lesion than with the more radical concept of pathology as a dynamic process. López Piñero has characterized these doctors, who simply asserted that dysfunction must be in the spinal cord, as 'functional localizers'.[38]

In *An Inquiry concerning that disturbed state of the vital functions usually denominated constitutional irritation* of 1826[39] Benjamin Travers, a surgeon at St Thomas's Hospital who had been educated at the home of Astley Cooper, picked out 'pain, unattended by any other sign of inflammation' as one of three categories of 'local irritation'.[40] Tic douloureux was attributed to 'a remote local irritation unattended by inflammation'.[41] Both the term and the concept of irritation were taken from Broussais. Travers's writing concurs with Cullen and Bichat in the attention paid to the condition of the tissues receiving perceptual stimuli:

> It is probable that...the operation of pain upon the system varies both with the character of the pain, and the state of the system...the nervous system excited by fever, or enfeebled by sickness of any kind, would receive impressions of pain widely different from those transmitted to it when overtaken by injury in a robust and healthy state.[42]

In addition to the physical condition of the tissues, the passions and imagination could distort sensibility and give rise to error. Travers used the expression 'sympathetic irritability' for sensibility 'deranged through the medium of the mind'.[43]

Tate's *A Treatise on Hysteria* of 1829 explored the relations between the moral realm, the uterus and the spinal cord in some detail in his discussion of the aetiology of the chronic, left-sided pains of hysteria.[44] Irritation was localized in the spinal cord, presumably reflecting the influence of Bell and Magendie's recent work. Tate was actually most precise: 'the upper dorsal portion of the spinal marrow' was involved. He was well aware that there were no post mortem findings to support his view and stated that he had neither the skill nor the opportunity to seek such evidence, nonetheless:

> Certain I feel, that, were these disorders to be profoundly investigated by...extensive anatomical research...Hysteria would be proven to have a local habituation in the spinal marrow and its meninges.[45]

He recommended Bell or Brodie to devote their careers to this task.

Tate considered the view that there might be 'some cause of mental inquietude at the bottom of an hysterical attack' in some detail:

> We know very well, how ready some young ladies are to be thought persons of high sensibility, and marvellously retentive of affecting events. When one of these has been lingering on under an unsuccessful treatment, month after month, it is frequently put to

her, with a sagacious, penetrating look, whether 'she has not something on her mind?'. At first, she invariably answers in the negative, and generally, in so answering, speaks the truth. But as soon as the practitioner has departed, she sets about a reminiscence of all the grievances she has incurred, the tears she has shed, and the trials she has passed, within the last twelve months; in which she is materially assisted by the ingenious memory of her silly relations. At last, some petty disappointment, or the death of some friend, far or near, is fixed upon, as having been a severe shock... the cause of the young lady's singular antics and of her various forms of illness, is settled at once.[46]

He rejected the idea that pains so disabling and severe 'take their rise from a lover's caprice' and asked how one would account for the good effects of medicines if the symptoms were of mental origin. He accepted that the mind is 'morbidly susceptible to impression of a painful kind' in such cases but believed disordered menstruation lay behind this. The proposed causal sequence was complex: irregular menstruation provoked a high state of excitement in the spinal marrow. The morbid susceptibility to painful impressions thus produced led to the chronic pains of hysteria. We can see how Tate seized on the work of Broussais and Bell to interpose a functionally deranged spinal cord between the uterus and the symptoms of Hysteria.

Thomas Pridgin Teale, whose son was the surgical collaborator of Clifford Allbutt in Leeds later in the century (see Chapter Six below), made use of spinal irritation to redefine and extend the meaning of the term neuralgia in *A Treatise on Neuralgic Diseases, dependent upon irritation of the spinal marrow and ganglia of the sympathetic nerve* (1830). In the opening pages he argued that the neuralgias

> have too often been regarded as actual diseases of those nervous filaments which are the immediate seat of the neuralgia instead of being considered as symptomatic of disease in the larger nervous masses from which those filaments are derived [i.e. spinal cord][47]

In support of his view he emphasized the new physical sign – small areas of spinal tenderness known as Player's spots – to be found in all cases of neuralgia. Teale described the clinical presentation of spinal irritation:

> severe and constant pain in one or both hypochondria...ceasing after lying down...endures for several years...attended with much constitutional disturbance [e.g. headache and neck pain]...the

depression in many cases is excessive...associated with menorrhagia, leucorrhoea, dysmenorrhoea and constipation.[48]

The contrast between local and constitutional disorder and the intimate relationship between spine and uterus were themes developed by others, notably Thomas Addison.

Addison's *Observations on the disorders of females connected with uterine irritation* of 1830[49] was a transcript of a lecture he had delivered a few years earlier. By 1830 he had been an Assistant Physician at Guy's Hospital for six years. *Observations* is of interest here for a number of reasons. It includes a careful definition of irritation and discussion of the perplexing topic of local versus generalized (constitutional) causes and effects in disease. It places the local pains of hysteria on an equal footing with the more spectacular hysterical paroxysms and attributes both to uterine irritation mediated by an obscure functional disturbance of the nervous system. Finally, moral causes are proposed for pain without lesion. Addison positions his lecture in opposition to Abernethy's recent account of the 'constitutional origin of local diseases'.[50] He argues that hysteria, far from being a constitutional disorder, has a local origin in irritation of the uterus and nervous system. Irritation, for Addison, lecturing in the 1820s, is 'a term in common use, to signify a disturbance in the endowments or functions of a part independent of either actual inflammation or organic lesion.'[51] Uterine irritation reveals its presence as irregular or painful menstruation and white vaginal discharge. The predisposing causes include nervous temperament (or constitutional irritability), sedentary and luxurious habits, late hours and passions of the mind. The exciting (or precipitating) cause is 'venereal excitement of every kind', notably 'imprudence during the menstrual period'.[52] The effect of uterine irritation was hysterical paroxysms and local pains. The most serious, prominent and interesting of the pains were those 'which attack the abdominal viscera, as these are repeatedly mistaken for inflammation'.[53] Addison listed six varieties of abdominal pain, the most common of which was 'a pain seated under the left mamma'. These pains are chronic, unaccompanied by fever and associated with tenderness on palpation: 'it may be called a general neuralgia of the abdomen'.[54]

Turning to specific case histories, Addison considered the state of the nervous system in hysteria. After dismissing altered nutrition, circulation or inflammation as aetiological factors he settled for

a morbid state of the nervous system generally, which...may be said to depend on some inscrutable change...independent of appreciable derangement either of structure or of vascular action.[55]

Thus invisible, functional derangement of the nervous system was interposed between uterus and symptom in hysteria, rather like in Tate's model.

A mixing of the thought of Bell and Broussais is quite apparent in this passage from Darwall's *An Essay on Spinal and Cerebral Irritation* of 1830:

> Mr Bell...in analysing the functions of different parts of the nervous system,...has clearly shewn that there are two portions, one of which bestows sensation, and the other the power of motion. The only part in which they can be separated by dissection is the spinal column...It is now much more generally acknowledged than formerly, that functional must precede organic diseases, and consequently, if the nervous system preside over and govern function, this same system must, in very many instances, be first affected...Of the nature of the irritation,...dissection cannot afford us any information, inasmuch as patients rarely die from maladies of this kind, till the functional has passed into organic disease. But I am inclined to believe, that in most cases there is some irregularity in the local circulation – that there is frequently congestion, and it may be conceived that it will sometimes proceed into acute or chronic inflammation.[56]

Darwall's essay is notable for other reasons. He, like Addison, mentions the distinction between local pains and other hysterical affections, such as palpitations or dyspnoea, among patients suffering spinal and cerebral irritation. The lengthy discussion of one case offers a closer look at Darwall's approach to pain without lesion. A 22-year-old woman

> had suffered from considerable depression of spirits for several months, when to this, pain in the side, stiffness in the back of the neck, palpitation of the heart, and dyspnoea, succeeded.[57]

The evidence for a disorder of the nervous system at the root of these various bodily symptoms is the predominance of mental symptoms verging on insanity: 'kindness is overlooked, or perversely misinterpreted; suspicions are entertained, the most unfounded and the most irrational.'[58] The local pains are also unaccompanied by inflammation and relieved by bedrest. These features are seen as typical of nervous pain. Darwall advocates moral management in addition to materia medica in such cases. He explains that moral management offers a way between the Scylla of an entirely conservative approach to 'an imaginary disease which it is useless to contend with, and impossible to overcome' and the Charybdis of charlatanism 'constantly attending, promising everything.'[59] The question as to what sort of doctor might be best equipped to treat patients with this functional nervous disorder is briefly raised and Darwall makes the case for a physician.

So a wide range of influences are at play in this text: Bell has drawn attention to the spinal cord, Broussais has offered a speculative functionalism, while the emphasis on the predominance of mental over somatic symptoms and advocacy of moral management remind us of Falret and Georgets' work. Interestingly Brodie is quoted approvingly and at length as the British authority on such conditions, and it is to his life and work that we now turn.

## 5. Brodie and Swan –
## Two Surgeons at the limits of Pathological Anatomy.

To understand how Benjamin Brodie came to be an expert on chronic pain, joint disease, neuralgia and hysteria, a list of conditions that look rather disparate today, it is important to remember that in the 1820s nerve pain and joint pain were both usually lesionless and were only just becoming distinguishable. The clear split between rheumatology and neurology was more than 60 years in the future. This is admirably illustrated by Scudamore's *Treatise on the nature and cure of rheumatism with observations on rheumatic neuralgia and on spasmodic neuralgia, or tic douloureux* of 1827.[60] The author claims this to be the first book-length account of rheumatism. In this text chronic rheumatism, sciatica, lumbago and tic douloureux were grouped together as chronic pains without inflammation and unaccompanied by fever. A number of case histories reveal how very difficult it was to distinguish one from another. This is the context that made Brodie's clinical acumen so exceptional in its day.

A lively biographical sketch of Benjamin Brodie is to be found in Bettany's *Eminent Doctors*.[61] Brodie studied anatomy in London under Abernethy and Wilson, and became a pupil of Sir Everard Home at St George's Hospital, between 1801 and his appointment as demonstrator in anatomy at Wilson's school in Great Windmill Street in 1805. At Windmill Street he lectured alongside Wilson until Bell's appointment there in 1812. He was appointed Assistant Surgeon at St George's Hospital in 1808, continuing his work there until 1840. He was at the top of the British surgical profession by the early 1820s, being Professor of Comparative Anatomy & Physiology at the Royal College of Surgeons and surgeon to Kings George IV and William IV. *The Lancet*, cited by Bettany, described him as a 'physician–surgeon' rather than an operating-surgeon; apparently he gave literally thousands of 'one guinea' private opinions over the course of his career. His particular area of expertise was distinguishing between joint disease, neuralgias and hysteria at the bedside, thus much of his clinical experience was focused precisely on pain and the question of presence or absence of lesion. This is quite clear from the opening passages of *Lectures Illustrative of certain Local Nervous Affections*, published in 1837,[62] near his retirement, but available in periodical form at least seven years earlier and delivered verbally before then.

The 'Advertisement' preceding the main body of this short monograph is devoted to espousing the pedagogic advantages of organizing a surgical book around symptoms rather than pathology, the reverse of the French method. This comes as a surprise at first, given that Brodie was very impressed by Bichat and that his 1818 book *On the pathology and surgery of diseases of the joints*[63] was firmly based on clinicopathological correlation. However, I shall be arguing that Brodie offers the clearest example of a surgeon, steeped in the new clinical method from France, who confronted and explored the limitations of, and exceptions to, that approach. The *Lectures* are precisely about symptoms, usually pains, unaccompanied by post-mortem lesions. The case vignette which introduces the lectures describes a clinical conundrum that was of pressing concern:

> A middle aged lady, who had been exposed during a considerable period of time to the operation of great mental anxiety, complained of a constant and severe pain, which she referred to a spot, about 3 or 4 inches in diameter, in the situation of the false ribs. Besides this she was subject to fits, apparently connected with hysteria, and was otherwise in a very impaired state of health. Under these circumstances she died, and on examining the body after death, particular attention was paid to the side to which the pain had been referred. No morbid appearances could be detected in it...Now such a case as this is by no means uncommon. It is only one of many which might be adduced in proof of this proposition, namely, that the natural sensations of a part may be increased, diminished, or otherwise perverted, although no disease exists in it which our senses are able to detect either before or after death.[64]

Brodie invokes disorder of the nervous system to account for such cases of pain apparently without lesion. Three distinct scenarios are elaborated in the book. In the first, the pain turns out to have an obvious lesion in the nervous system proximal to the area where the pain is felt, i.e. the pain is at a distance from lesion and can be explained by detailed knowledge of neuroanatomy. For example, pain in the little finger on striking the elbow is understood through an appreciation of the course of the ulnar nerve.[65] The second clinical scenario is pain at a spatial distance from lesion where there is 'no direct communication between the nerves of the parts affected that will afford a reasonable explanation of the occurrence of the sympathetic pain.'[66] An example might be pain in the foot plus dyspepsia or pain in the foot plus internal piles. In such cases

> in all probability it is in the brain itself that the communication is made, the impression first being transmitted to the sensorium, and from thence reflected to the nerves of the part which is secondarily affected. If you dissect the brain...you will find it splitting into fibres, passing in various directions, many of which...connecting even the most distant convolutions of the cerebrum with each other...we may..suppose that an impression on one part of the body should, by means of these communicating fibres, produce a disordered sensation in another part.[67]

Thus Brodie invokes the detailed internal anatomy of the brain itself as the substrate for a process he calls 'reflection' by which he explains this type of pain at a distance from lesion. It seems unlikely that this indicates any interest on his part in Marshall Hall's contemporary writings; he is coining the term independently here. Brodie did not elaborate 'reflection' beyond this single use of the word in this text and it clearly does not refer to a sensori-motor arc.

One very telling assumption in Brodie's thought is that any lesion anywhere in the body will do to account for an otherwise inexplicable pain. Only when the whole body is free of structural lesion in life and death does he begin to consider a constitutional, rather than local, disorder as cause for pain. However, in the third clinical scenario Brodie encountered – local pains in association with classical symptoms of hysteria (such as fits or aphonia) and in the absence of any lesion – he was forced to accept the localized pain as a feature of the generalized, constitutional disorder of hysteria . He called such pain a 'local hysterical affection'. Two of the three lectures in the book were devoted to it.

Thus Brodie seems to have been the first to draw a clear distinction between neuralgic pain, with a local cause somewhere in the nervous system, and hysterical pain of more diffuse origin. This was to prove of considerable heuristic value.

Brodie offers a detailed account of the characteristics of local hysteria.[68] He found it among the female patients he saw in private practice much more than among hospital inpatients. Four fifths of all the supposed joint disease of upper class women is local hysteria, he claimed. It is rarely seen in men. The usual age of onset is just after puberty. The symptom tends to come on gradually and may be precipitated by moral causes or by the debilitating effects of long illness. Menstruation is sometimes irregular. Once sleep is initiated it continues uninterrupted, in contrast to the pain of organic joint pathology. The pain drags on for years but no serious pathology, such as abscess or joint deformation, appears. On bedside examination there are a number of subtle signs that point to the diagnosis of local hysteria. The whole limb is painful, rather than certain joints. The application of pressure to many parts of the body provokes screams. There is more reaction to pinching of the skin than to weightbearing at the joint: 'If you pinch the skin...the patient complains more than when you forcibly squeeze the head of the thigh-bone into the socket of the acetabulum.'[69] The more the patient focuses attention on the examination, the more exaggerated the reaction to pain. There is no wasting of muscles but there may be some swelling of extremities due to disuse and immobility.

Turning to the pathology of hysteria Brodie was clearly a 'functional localizer':

> We cannot doubt that its locality is in the nervous system. This is sufficiently demonstrated by the character of the symptoms themselves. Dissection...affords us little assistance here; at least we derive from it only negative information.[70]

He described three post mortems he had conducted himself, in which he had paid particular attention to the painful part and the appearance of the nervous system. No structural disorganization was to be found. Despite these negative findings Brodie expects that 'imperfect development of the nervous system' due to 'injudicious management in the early part of life' and some hereditary influence produces the vulnerability to hysteria. The disorder is then precipitated by moral or physical causes. Among the former he mentions anxiety or 'a disappointment' while the latter include weakness due to loss of blood.

Brodie advocates a mixture of moral and physical management for established cases. Tonics and antispasmodics should be combined with exercise and light, diverting occupation. Tedium and bloodletting must be avoided. The first because in boredom 'the mind is...thrown back upon itself, brooding over imaginary misfortunes, and creating for itself objects of anxiety' and the second because bloodletting increases debility. Brodie states that he does not favour counter-irritation techniques, such as moxa, because they fix the patient's attention on the part that they are already overconcerned about. However, a slim volume by a J.T.Boyle, published in 1826,[71] suggests that Brodie's actions belied his words. In this book Boyle claims to have accepted a number of referrals of patients with chronic, painful joint conditions from Brodie for the application of moxa as a treatment of last resort. The use of Brodie's famous name to legitimize Boyle's therapeutics was no doubt strategic but it is unlikely that Boyle simply lied about the referrals (see Rey[72] for an account of moxa in French medical writing of 1820s). Finally, Brodie warns against amputating for pain alone, as did Bell.

We have seen that Brodie only admitted hysteria as a cause of localized pain with reluctance. I shall now describe some of the work of Joseph Swan, a surgeon about one decade junior to Brodie, who went further still in resisting generalized origins for local pains. It will be argued that Swan was an arch-proponent of the new anatomoclinical method who described the extensive impact of localized, structural lesion. An explanation for his extreme position will be offered, based on his professional biography.

Swan's *Treatise on Diseases and Injuries of the Nerves* (1834)[73] was an enlarged and updated version of his Jacksonian Prize essay of 1819. It was devoted to nervous pain, as the titles of the first two chapters make clear: 'Of painful affections of nerves in general','Of painful affections in particular nerves'. The competing claims of local and constitutional explanations for nervous pain were reviewed:

> The pain in many cases has been so entirely confined to one nerve, and attended with so little apparent disorder of the system generally, as to have led to the belief of its having been entirely local. But, on the contrary, since [division of nerve] has proved so often unsuccessful, the conclusion that the disease is constitutional has been as generally adopted.[74]

Swan went on to outline interactions between irritated viscera, brain irritation and localized nervous pains in similar terms to Broussais and Bell. He argued that although localized chronic pain can have ill effects on the brain this does not mean the pain is constitutional in origin:

> It is desirable to lean as little as possible to such suggestions, which

are the mere opinions of despair, and...tend to... prevent that due attention to pathological researches which may extend the means of relief.[75]

In a number of detailed case histories he showed how minor structural lesions could have profound, generalized influence on the sufferer. He particularly drew attention to the effects of partial division of peripheral nerves.

CASE 1[76]: Mrs E, aged 40. Cut her left thumb. Two weeks later, spasms of pain began all over the body 'as if her flesh was being pinched with hot irons...as if hot water was being poured down her back'. These continued for seven years with gradual improvement but still 'the mere carrying of an umbrella two hours produced sensations all over her body, as if needles were running into her, also restlessness, pain at the stomach and head-ache'. She died nine years after the accident but post mortem was refused. Nonetheless Swan attributed her chronic pain to the cut thumb.

CASE 2[77]: A 26 year old surgeon's wife from Lincolnshire. Cut her thumb with a breadknife. Pain for two years. Required large doses of opiates and was close to mental derangement because of the pain. Restored to perfect health by the amputation of the thumb.

CASE 3[78]: Miss Wilson, aged 23. Cut her left hand while peeling an orange. Over the next month pains in the hand, arm, left breast, left face, neck, back of ear, left clavicle and right side of abdomen. Seven months later she complained of back pain and left-sided chest pain and became bedbound despite going to a seaside resort. Eighteen months later 'on making an examination of the spine, pressure on each side of the spinous processes of several of the vertebrae produced pain, and percussion with a key made it very severe'. She now developed left knee pain. Her condition was unchanged some eleven years after the injury. 'It is worthy of remark, that the left half of the body seems to have suffered throughout by the accident, and the right very little.' Swan again attributed all the symptoms over the 11 years of disability to the minor structural lesion of a digital nerve which he presented as a Plate in the book.

In a later chapter on the sympathetic nerve Swan suggests that one major function of this structure is communication between distant parts of the body. In health it underlies the coordination of bodily functions, while in disease it conveys the ill effects of injury very widely. If the 'constitutional irritation' provoked by a local injury is great enough it may cause death. He describes the post mortem appearances of the sympathetic ganglia in a child who died a few days after a modest burn. The ganglia were redder than expected, indicating to Swan their role in propagating fatal irritation all over the body.[79]

It seems rather perverse to us that Swan should be satisfied with a trivial lesion of a digital nerve as an explanation for a decade of multiple, disabling pains all over the body. But what was at stake for him were the tenets of the new anatomoclinical method. The whole thrust of this programme was to match symptom and lesion, even if the lesion was at a distance from the pain and the pain was out of all proportion to the lesion. Swan was reluctant to concede defeat on this and fall back on old concepts such as Brunonian debility or asthenia. In cases of pain where there was absolutely no disease anywhere in the body he accepted that tonics and purgatives might be valuable as traditional medical treatment for debility but had grave reservations. He argued that lesionless pain was sometimes a functional brain disorder and opiates or tonics had the potential to worsen the condition:

> If the seat of the disorder be in the brain, it is a serious question whether the quantities of opium, ether, and stimulants, so frequently had recourse to in these cases, have not the tendency to increase the malady, and whether the moral treatment of the patient would not be more likely to effect a salutary change.[80]

This nod towards moral management warns us against reading Swan as rejecting pain psychology altogether in the light of the growing appreciation of neuro-anatomy. He actually devoted a book to the interaction of mind and body in the 1850s in which he explicitly stated that the passions alone may cause pain:

'Anxiety and fear may convey irritation from the mind to the whole brain or particular centres, as those of the nerves of the limbs, so as to impair their activity and produce pain'.[81]

Why was Swan an even stronger advocate of local causes for local pains than Brodie? At first sight they had almost identical backgrounds and interests. Both had begun their careers as brilliant students of surgery in the London teaching hospitals. Both had a special interest in painful conditions. Both wrote 'psychological' books on retirement in the 1850s (see Brodie's *Psychological Inquiries* of 1855[82]) in which they tackled the relationship between mind and body. But there was an important biographical difference. Brodie was an active clinician throughout his career while Swan was more talented as a dissector. From 1827 to 1870 he dissected humans and animals, and performed animal vivisection, full-time in a converted billiard room at his London home. He lived in relative obscurity, relying on Astley Cooper, Abernethy and others for human corpses, sent to him annually in the guise of a Christmas hamper. This detachment from the complexities of clinical work with chronic pain patients allowed him to settle for rather weak explanations for the baffling phenomenology of hysterical females that Brodie, Addison and others encountered daily.

### 6. The continuing British debate about Surgical Hysteria in the 1860s

Micale[83] has rightly drawn attention to the historical neglect of a British tradition of texts on 'surgical hysteria'. In response to this I should like to leap chronologically some 25 years to the 1860s to examine how Brodie's 'local hysteria' was taken up by two London teaching hospital surgeons. In the writings of Hilton and Skey we encounter the ongoing debate between clinicians and purer anatomists over pain without lesion.

John Hilton's lectures of 1860–62, delivered in his new capacity as Professor of Anatomy and Surgery at the Royal College of Surgeons, were the result of over 30 years' anatomical study and about 20 years' clinical surgical experience, all at Guy's Hospital. He had been appointed Demonstrator in Anatomy after just four years as a medical student and spent the decade 1828–38 performing meticulous dissections which were then copied in wax by Joseph Towne. After this prolonged period of anatomical study he mixed clinical work as a surgeon and lecturing in Anatomy. The lectures to the Royal College represent the summit of his career and were published in 1863 under the title *On the influence of mechanical and physiological rest in the treatment of accidents and surgical diseases, and the diagnostic value of pain.*[84] Under the abbreviated title *Rest and Pain* this text was very widely read over the next few decades. I shall present a close reading of the 'clinical remarks on pain as a symptom of disease' and contrast Hilton's views on lesionless pain with those of a contemporaneous surgeon at St Bartholomew's Hospital, F.C.Skey. I shall argue that the divergence between these authors on the topic almost recapitulates that between Swan and Brodie some 25 years earlier, and for the same reason.

Hilton began by loosening the quartet of signs and symptoms of inflammation: pain is very often found in isolation and is not a reliable marker of inflammation or true surgical disease, i.e. structural lesion. Calor, not dolor, is closest to a pathognomonic feature of inflammation. Pain without inflammation 'must be looked upon as caused by an exalted sensitiveness of the nerves of the part...depending upon a cause situated remotely from the part where it is felt'. It results 'from some direct nervous communication passing between the part where the pains are expressed and the real and remotely situated cause of the pain'. He called it 'sympathetic pain'.[85] Note that Broussais, the French physician, and Hilton, a surgeon, started from similar but distinct observations on the relationship between pain and inflammation. While Broussais held that pain precedes inflammatory lesion in the chronic phlegmasias, Hilton here reported that pain is at a spatial rather than temporal distance from structural lesion in many surgical diseases. Broussais's solution had been to invoke an invisible process, irritation, while Hilton set himself the task of discovering 'what association of nerves will explain this [sympathetic] pain?'[86] This was an important difference between the schools of *médecine physiologique* and pathological anatomy. Hilton did not entertain the possibility of pain without structural lesion and devoted great energy to discovering what one might call 'the anatomy of sympathy'. Like Swan, Hilton was vehemently opposed to the attribution of local pain to constitutional disturbances. He saw explanations such as rheumatism, gout, inherited weakness, etc., as words concealing medical ignorance. His approach was summarized thus:

> external pain, or pain upon the surface of the body, if properly appreciated, may be considered as an external sign of some distant derangement. If the pain persists – if it does not depend on any transient cause - it becomes necessary to seek the precise position of the pain; and as soon as we recognise the precise position of the pain, we are enabled, by a knowledge of the distribution of the nerve or nerves of that part, to arrive at once at the only rational suggestion as to what nerve is the exponent of the symptom. By following centripetally the course of that nerve, and bearing in mind its relation to surrounding structures, we shall, in all probability, be able to reach the original, the producing cause of pain, and, consequently, to adopt the correct diagnosis.[87]

An important question comes to mind with this quote. It is the suspicion that Hilton might have been describing an ideal of how a surgeon would wish to proceed, using applied anatomy to the full to explain the clinical conundrum of pain as an isolated symptom. How often could this ideal, perhaps born in the dissecting room, actually be met in practice? Hilton's case reports illustrate some triumphs of his anatomical analysis of sympathetic pains.

Hilton offered several case reports of lower abdominal pain due to disease of the spine and, in a clear response to Brodie's work, proposed an 'explanation of hysterical pains in the hip or knee joint'. He argued that the sacral ganglia of the sympathetic nerve supply the ovaries and part of the uterus and are connected to the great sciatic nerve:

> If nerves in the ovaries or the uterus be in a state of irritation, that irritation can be conducted to these sacral nerves...and then, in accordance with the generally received law of distribution of nervous influence, irritation or pain may be manifested at the other peripheral or articular end of the same nerve. Hence it may be expressed [at the knee or hip joints].[88]

Here we see Hilton offer a fully argued anatomical explanation for 'Brodie's hip', the classic instance of 'local hysteria'.

The conflict between the patient and surgeons' perceptions of the site of the lesion could be a recipe for dissatisfaction as Hilton acknowledged:

> Patients judge of the position of their own disease...by the situation of the most prominent painful symptoms...; whilst we surgeons, relying upon our knowledge of the true cause of the symptoms, judge of the seat of the disease by a just interpretation of the symptoms through the medium of normal anatomy.[89]

One case was a man with disease of the spine manifested as abdominal pain.[90] The patient could not accept this opinion and secretly sought a second opinion from Brodie, who agreed with Hilton's judgement. Both had advised rest but the patient was non-compliant and by now doctor–patient relations were becoming strained. Hilton described the patient as 'monstrously conceited, thinking himself right and everybody else wrong'. Given that he 'could not be controlled in his own house', admission to Guy's was arranged. As he was beginning to recover with rest he took his own discharge against medical advice. When he fully recovered some time later Hilton learned that the patient attributed his relief to 'hydrotherapy and homeopathy' rather than to the surgeon's interventions. Hilton's conclusion to this tale of conflicting interpretations of pain between doctor and patient was to modestly point out to his audience: 'It so happens, gentlemen, sometimes, that we do not get the degree of credit which perhaps belongs to us'.

To summarize, Hilton, ever the anatomist, answered the problem of pain without lesion with pain at a distance from structural lesion.

He was squarely in the tradition of pathological anatomy as he tried to elucidate an anatomy of sympathy, very much as Joseph Swan had done 25 years before. I have raised the possibility that Hilton's explanation of all pain without lesion as 'referred pain' from structural pathology might have been an ideal rather than a reality. I shall now present a monograph by Skey, a contemporary of Hilton, which supports this historical scepticism.

Skey dedicated his 1867 monograph on *Hysteria*[91] to Brodie. Taking his cue from Brodie's observations of young women with joint pains Skey stated 'pain alone, which consists in an exalted nervous sensibility, does not constitute what we strictly understand by the term disease'.[92] For Skey 'Real disease is the exception' in the practice of clinical surgery.[93] To understand what Skey was saying it is worth pausing to review his notion of 'real disease'. Like Hilton, he separated the inflammatory quartet. Redness, as an isolated finding, points to congestion rather than inflammation while pain alone implies nervous disorder rather than disease of the vasculature (i.e. congestion/inflammation) (Lecture 1). While local inflammations have local causes, local pains for the most part have central causes 'the effects of which are exhibited in remote parts of the body'.[94] The central cause of many pains is irritation of the brain and spinal cord – hysteria. So Skey was arguing, in contradiction to Hilton, that most pain without lesion is due to a central functional derangement rather than local surgical disease at a distance from the pain.

Skey specified the type of hysteria that is the province of the surgeon. The symptoms of general hysteria, such as globus, crying, palpitations and polyuria are best managed by physicians while local hysteria or surgical hysteria, that is, pain or fixed contractures, should be managed by surgeons.[95] Skey distinguished between the pain of local hysteria and that of 'simple neuralgia' by means of the spatial distribution of the pains on the surface of the body:

> In Neuralgia the disease is placed on a recognised nerve, and a person is said to have Neuralgia of a given nerve, such as the frontal, mental or digital. In Hysteria any locality may be affected without reference to the distribution of nerves.[96]

He also favoured some sort of mental aetiology for hysteria: 'It is a very interesting question to investigate how far the functions of the mind are involved in hysteric disease...In cases of local pain...it seems difficult to identify the evil with that part of the brain which we believe to be the seat of the mind' but, he concludes, such a causal relation does exist.

Taken together, these views on the distinctive spatialization of neurogenic pain and hysterical pain of mental origin were most influential on Charcot, as Micale[97] has highlighted. The closing words of the book support this: 'finally, in considering the entire phenomena of hysteric affections, it is difficult to deny their relation to the mind, which appears to exercise some mysterious or occult influence over them.'[98] The case history of an 18-year-old woman who, for many years, had suffered stomach pain after eating provides an insight into the kind of clinical experience that led Skey to this conclusion:

> On entering the drawing room, I heard the sound of suffering from an adjoining room... Having intruded myself into the room somewhat unexpectedly by its occupants, I saw this young lady in a condition of great suffering, in the upright position, leaning her head on her mother's shoulder, and sobbing painfully.

He insisted on interviewing the girl alone:

> I spoke of her home and the scenery around it, of which I described the general characters, and enlarged on the beauty of the neighbourhood, the lovely rides and excursions, etc.,... during the few minutes which this conversation occupied she was to all appearance entirely free from pain... I then changed the subject by saying, 'I think your pain has flown away,' when she immediately resumed her crying fit, and sobbed as before.[99]

He thus reached the diagnosis of Hysteria. One interesting feature of Skey's report is the way the competing perceptions of patient and surgeon clash. The surgeon relies on 'appearance' rather than the verbalized subjective complaint of the pain patient. This supports Foucault's generalizations about the priority of the 'medical gaze' in the clinical method of the century. This patient was as dissatisfied with the outcome as Hilton's 'monstrously conceited' male patient had been when told that the problem did not coincide in space with his pain. And it was not only patients who did not welcome the opinions of these anatomoclinicians. Sometimes the relatives thought little of the doctor's conclusions too, as this next case illustrates.

A 24-year-old woman who had been horizontal in her bedroom for five years due to back pain sought Skey's opinion after multiple consultations with other doctors. On examination he found pain and tenderness precisely localized to the L2 vertebra but a mobile trunk. These he interpreted as classical stigmata of local hysteria. He told her father that the diagnosis was hysteria but 'failed to convince' and never saw the patient again.[100]

I should like to propose that the conclusions reached by Skey and Hilton about surgical hysteria almost exactly mirror the disagreement between Brodie and Swan years earlier. Once again we see the more theoretically oriented dissector advocating a 'pure' version of clinico-pathological correlation. For Swan and Hilton there must be a structural lesion corresponding to a local pain, the challenge is to find it and to explain the functional connection between symptom and disease in terms of applied anatomy. In contrast, Brodie and Skey, as busy surgical clinicians, in response to endless consultations with patients complaining of pain but apparently free of disease, more readily invoked the notion of a central nervous system dysfunction, Hysteria, at the root of pain without lesion.

## Summary

I have argued that Broussais's extension of the concept of lesion to include a temporal element, invisible irritation preceding the visible structural derangement of inflammation, was widely influential in France and Britain in this period. I tend to concur with Foucault's view that he 'saved' the new clinical method. A number of authors in Britain combined this speculative functionalism with Bell and Magendies' emphasis on the spinal roots to develop the notion of spinal irritation as a cause for pain without lesion – a move López Piñero has called 'functional localisation'. Yet, among the authors reviewed here, perhaps only Fourcade-Prunet and Broussais really grasped how radical a temporal, as well as spatial, appreciation of pathology could be in linking symptom and functional lesion. None of the British authors sought to explain issues such as the intermittent pattern of pain in tic douloureux, busy as they were using the new idea of an invisible lesion. In other words, I am suggesting that most seized on irritation at the visuospatial level, as explanation for symptoms apparently without lesion, while underemphasizing the dynamic or transitory potential of putative functional lesions. Charcot was to make more of this temporal element much later in the century.

The tension between local and generalized symptoms and pathologies runs through several of these texts, notably Addison, Darwall, Brodie and Swan. A reluctance to settle for a 'constitutional' explanation for local symptoms was at the heart of the new clinical method from France, even when this forced the clinician into quite extreme positions (such as Swan's attribution of a decade of disability to a tiny digital nerve injury, rather than accepting the symptoms as lesionless). One important nosological consequence of this struggle was the division of hysteria into local and more classical, generalized symptoms in the writings of Darwall, Addison and Brodie. This placing of chronic pains without lesion on an equal footing with the more spectacular motor manifestations of hysteria in the 1830s is at odds with one of Shorter's central arguments.[101] He insists that the 'quieter' sensory symptoms of hysteria were not 'upgraded' until after Charcot's work of the 1880s.

Far from heralding an era in which the findings of neuroanatomy and experimental physiology drowned out traditional sensitivity to 'pain psychology', I have found some textual evidence that Bell shared Broussais's interest in gastric irritation as an explanation for some lesionless pain in his mature clinical work of the early 1830s. It has also been shown that even a dedicated neuroanatomist like Swan was open to the ideas of pain of mental origin and moral management of some pain patients.

One final comment. There is very considerable overlap and agreement, among the authors surveyed, on the clinical picture of pain without structural lesion, while the terms used to name it varied a good deal: local irritation, sympathetic irritability, spinal irritation, nervous pain, neuralgic pain or local hysteria. The clinical features are most fully collated in Brodie's writing, but the left-sided predominance of such pain, the negligible mortality from it, the female preponderance, risk of opiate dependence and several other characteristics are repeated from one author to the next. Over the course of the book I shall continue to compare case histories to see how historically invariant, or otherwise, the clinical presentation of pain without lesion has been. One might expect the clinical syndrome to change over time as techniques for detecting lesions in vivo and post mortem improved. This technological development would render more and more previously apparently lesionless pains organic, leaving a purer residuum of patients for whom chronic pain had perhaps a psychological basis. However, my historical research tends to show that the symptoms, complications and prognosis of chronic pain without lesion have remained remarkably stable over time.

## Notes

1 Foucault, 1973, ch 10, *The Birth of the Clinic: an archaeology of medical perception.*

2 Bynum, 1994, 45, *Science and the Practice of Medicine in the Nineteenth Century.*

3 Foucault, 1973, ch 10, *The Birth of the Clinic: an archaeology of*

*medical perception.*

4  Broussais, 1826, *A Treatise on Physiology Applied to Pathology.*

5  *Ibid.*, 26–28.

6  *Ibid.*, 48–49.

7  *Ibid.*, 111.

8  *Ibid.*, 111–12.

9  *Ibid.*, 125.

10  *Ibid.*, 126.

11  *Ibid.*, 129.

12  *Ibid.*, 190.

13  *Ibid.*, 198–99.

14  Fourcade-Prunet, 1826, *Maladies Nerveuses des auteurs, raportées a l'irritation de l'encéphale, des nerfs cérébro-rachidiens et splanchniques, avec ou sans inflammation*

15  *Ibid.*, 103.

16  Merskey & Spear, 1967, 7, *Pain: psychological and psychiatric aspects.*

17  Morris, 1991, 4–5, *The Culture of Pain.*

18  Bell, 1806, *Essays on the Anatomy of Expression.*

19  Bynum, 1976, 15–16, *Varieties of Cartesian experience in early-nineteenth-century neurophysiology*

20  Bell, 1806, 98, *Essays on the Anatomy of Expression.*

21  *Ibid.*, 118.

22  *Ibid.*, 161–2.

23  Bell, 1811, *Idea of a New Anatomy of the Brain*

24  Cranefield, 1974, *The Way In and the Way Out: François Magendie, Charles Bell and the roots of the spinal nerves.*

25  Rice, 1987, *The Bell–Magendie–Walker controversy.*

26  Rey, 1993, 207–8, *History of Pain*

27  Bell, 1836, *The Nervous System of the Human Body.*

28  *Ibid.*, 9.

29  *Ibid.*, 356.

30  *Ibid.*, 350.

31  *Ibid.*, 364.

32  *Ibid.*

33  *Ibid.*, 365.

34  *Ibid.*, 366.

35  *Ibid.*, 368–9.

36  López Piñero, 1983, 63–4, *Historical Origins of the Concept of Neurosis.*

37  Shorter, 1992, ch 2, *From Paralysis to Fatigue: a history of psychosomatic illness in the modern era.*

38  López Piñero, 1983, 53, *Historical Origins of the Concept of Neurosis.*

39 Travers, 1826, *An Inquiry concerning that disturbed state of the vital functions usually denominated constitutional irritation.*

40 *Ibid.,* 35.

41 *Ibid.,* 36.

42 *Ibid.,* 57.

43 *Ibid.,* 14.

44 Tate, 1829, 42, *A Treatise on Hysteria.*

45 *Ibid.,* 132

46 *Ibid.,* 130–131.

47 Teale, 1830, 2, *A Treatise on Neuralgic Diseases, dependent upon irritation of the spinal marrow and ganglia of the sympathetic nerve.*

48 *Ibid.,* 10–11.

49 Addison, 1830, *Observations on the disorders of females connected with uterine irritation*

50 *Ibid.,* 9.

51 *Ibid.,* 10–11.

52 *Ibid.,* 13.

53 *Ibid.,* 21

54 *Ibid.,* 27.

55 *Ibid.,* 68–9

56 Darwall, 1830, 189–91, *An Essay on spinal and cerebral irritation.*

57 *Ibid.,* 201.

58 *Ibid.,* 205.

59 *Ibid.,* 208.

60 Scudamore, 1827, *A Treatise on the nature and cause of rheumatism with observations on rheumatic neuralgia and on spasmodic neuralgia, or Tic Douloureux.*

61 Bettany, 1885, *Eminent Doctors: their lives and their work.*

62 Brodie, 1837, *Lectures Illustrative of certain local nervous affections.*

63 Brodie, 1818, *Pathological and surgical observations on diseases of the joints.*

64 Brodie, 1837, 1–2, *Lectures Illustrative of certain local nervous affections.*

65 *Ibid.,* 3.

66 *Ibid.,* 14.

67 *Ibid.,* 14–15.

68 *Ibid.,* 36–46.

69 *Ibid.,* 38.

70 *Ibid.,* 66.

71 Boyle, 1826, *A Treatise on a modified application of moxa, in the treatment of stiff and contracted joints.*

72 Rey, 1993, 155–6, *History of Pain.*

73 Swan, 1834, *A Treatise on diseases and injuries of the nerves*
74 *Ibid.*, 3.
75 *Ibid.*, 23.
76 *Ibid.*, 124–7.
77 *Ibid.*, 127–8.
78 *Ibid.*, 129–41.
79 *Ibid.*, 302–4.
80 *Ibid.*, 56.
81 Swan, 1854, 74, *The Brain in relation to the mind.*
82 Brodie, 1855, *Psychological Inquiries.*
83 Micale, 1989, *Hysteria and its historiography: a review of past and present writings.*
84 Hilton, 1863, *On the influence of mechanical and physiological rest in the treatment of accidents and surgical diseases, and the diagnostic value of pain.*
85 *Ibid.*, 68–9.
86 *Ibid.*, 69.
87 *Ibid.*, 70.
88 *Ibid.*, 224.
89 *Ibid.*, 70.
90 *Ibid.*, 70–72.
91 Skey, 1867, *Hysteria.*
92 *Ibid.*, 48.
93 *Ibid.*, 45.
94 *Ibid.*, 40.
95 *Ibid.*, 51–2.
96 *Ibid.*, 64–5.
97 Micale, 1990b, *Charcot and the idea of hysteria in the male: gender, mental science, and medical diagnosis in late nineteenth-century France.*
98 Skey, 1867, 107, *Hysteria.*
99 *Ibid.*, 92–3.
100 *Ibid.*, 77–9.
101 Shorter, 1992, 150, *From Paralysis to Fatigue: a history of psychosomatic illness in the modern era.*

# 3

## Gemeingefühl

## German Romanticism, Cenesthesis and Subjective Pain: 1794–1846

The next group of texts are from early nineteenth-century 'Germany'[1]. They differ from the primary sources examined here thus far, having been written by professors in universities rather than active clinicians. Most of the work was on the normal physiology of humans and animals; patients with unexplained symptoms were not the foremost daily concern of these academics. When they wrote about pain, they mostly described the pain of experimental, rather than pathological, conditions. Nevertheless, the writings of Müller, Weber and others loom large in standard histories of pain and I intend to make a number of rather unusual claims based on these writings.

It will be argued that pain was set apart from the senses of touch, taste, smell, vision and hearing and was subsumed within the concept of cenesthesis *(Gemeingefühl)* by many German authors between 1794 and 1894. Now cenesthesis is not a well-known concept in Anglophone medical writings. It means bodily feeling in the most diffuse and general sense. It can be contrasted with the special senses. Cenesthesis is something like a feeling tone or background subjective state of being. So long as pain was considered as part of cenesthesis it remained to one side of the rapid developments in the neurophysiology and psychology of sensation/perception in the second half of the century, exemplified by the work of Helmholtz. The lack of any putative receptor organ for pain (equivalent to the eye or ear) prior to von Frey's 'pain spots' of 1894 provides the most obvious explanation for this relative neglect, but it will be suggested that the conceptual distinction between cenesthesis and extracorporeal sensation also played a part. My argument follows Boring[2] who claimed that 'Von Frey in 1894 was most instrumental in getting pain out of the *Gemeingefühl*'. If these views can be confirmed then a major blow is dealt to those historians who have offered accounts of nineteenth-century pain physiology as reductionist neuroscience. I have in mind Merskey & Spear[3] and Morris[4] in particular. If pain was embedded in the Romantic notion of cenesthesis throughout the century then it lay outside the empirical 'biophysics' that the '1847 Group' and later researchers self-consciously strove towards (see Cranefield[5] and Tuchman[6] for good accounts of the 1847 manifesto of Helmholtz, du Bois-Reymond, Brücke and Ludwig). So long as pain was an aspect of bodily feeling in general it could not be reduced to a predictable response to a stimulus or lesion.

The second argument I shall propose is that sensations without external referents, notably subjective visual phenomena and subjective pain, were the observational basis of Müller's famous doctrine of specific nerve energies. This view is based on an interesting paper by Riese & Arrington[7]. To put it most sharply, it was auto-experimentation with subjective sensations, and not electrophysiological experiments, that gave rise to the doctrine depicted by some historians as the exemplar of a reductionist neuroscience. Far from reducing the open eighteenth-century concept of sensibility to a narrow scientific concept of sensation – a predictable response to a stimulus – Müller went out of his way to emphasize that sensation says more about the subject feeling it than about any stimulus provoking it.

The third and final purpose of this section is to show how lesionless pains were accounted for in terms of disordered cenesthesis in the writings of two German Romantic psychiatrists, Reil and Feuchtersleben. I shall also suggest that pain without lesion was distinctly unproblematic for Müller.

To establish this rather complex series of claims the concept of cenesthesis will first be outlined and put in context. I shall demonstrate that many German authors throughout the century placed pain within it. A close reading of Müller's *Elements of Physiology* [8] and mention of his earlier physiological writings will be used to support the second argument. Finally, I offer a discussion of pain without lesion and cenesthesis in the writings of Reil, Feuchtersleben, Weber and Müller.

### 1. Pain and Cenesthesis

Attention has been drawn to the concept of cenesthesis by a number of historians of nineteenth-century sensory physiology and psychology, notably Boring[9], Schiller[10] and Starobinski.[11] Cenesthesis has several confusing synonyms, depending upon the language used by its advocates: *Gemeingefühl, sensibilité générale, cénesthésie,* coenaesthesia, common sensibility. It must be carefully distinguished from 'common sense' and the *sensorium commune*, both of which have much longer histories.

## J.C.Reil

'Cenesthesis' was first coined in 1794 in a doctoral thesis at the University of Halle, nominally by Hubner but thought to have been penned by J.C.Reil. Marx[12] gives biographical details of this fascinating man who coined the word 'psychiatry' as well as becoming the first professor of physiology at the newly-founded University of Berlin in 1810. In 1794 Reil had been professor of medicine at Halle for about six years.

His concept of cenesthesis depended upon a tripartite division of perception: perception of the state of one's own body, perception of extracorporeal objects and awareness of the activities of one's own mind. Cenesthesis was the first of these modes of perception and Reil included ten varieties of pain, as well as hunger and thirst, within the category. Although Descartes had proposed a similar tripartite division this was not Reil's inspiration. Rather, the appeal of the concept of cenesthesis in the context of German Romantic Psychiatry[13] must be briefly explained. It was consistent with Romantic concerns for unity, graded developmental hierarchy and the relation between an active perceiving subject (percipiens) and the material world. This is not the place to expand on these key themes in post-Kantian thought (for which see Rothschuh[14], Risse[15,16], Leary[17], Clarke & Jacyna[18] and Marx[19]). Suffice it to say that cenesthesis was the most elementary core experience of pure lived duration imaginable. It was the bedrock of a continuing notion of personal identity and integrity in the face of the torrent of fleeting thoughts of waking life and the repeated interruption that is sleep. Developmentally it was regarded as the first, and most primitive, of the three categories of perception to appear. A newborn baby, Reil argued, feels pain, hunger and thirst before it perceives external objects or becomes aware of its own mental activity. Note that for an empiricist the development of a human is the accumulation of percepts while for Reil the very nature of the percipiens changes over time.

### E. H. Weber

E. H. Weber certainly followed Reil in drawing a distinction between the sense of touch (extracorporeal sensation) and pain (cenesthesis). This is exemplified in the title and content of his monograph, published in 1846 but representing his thought since the early 1830s, *Der Tastsinn und das Gemeingefühl.*[20] In this text he contrasted touch, well localized in space and time and finely graded in intensity, with pain.[21] He saw pain as the result of overstimulation of any sensory

nerve by stimuli 'so intense that they not only stimulate the
nerve-endings, but also their trunks: pain is evoked, the faculty of
desire is excited in the mind, and calm reflection is prevented.'[22] A
good example of this would be photophobia, when light causes pain
by overstimulation of the retina.[23] He suggested that touch and pain
must involve different brain regions since etherization can affect one
without the other.[24] Perhaps the clearest wording of the contrast
Weber drew between cenesthesis and extracorporeal sensation is the
following:

> [Cenesthesis is] our ability to perceive our own sensory states, e.g.
> pain; this condition is therefore distinguished from our ability to
> have a sensation derived from an object distinct from our own
> sensory state itself, e.g. the sensation of a colour or a tone. This
> ability has therefore never been taken to be a typical sense modality.
> Rather...all our sensory nerves, under certain circumstances, can
> provide us with sensations of this kind.[25]

Most of Weber's 'experiments' were autoexperimentation
combined with introspection. For example, he described undergoing
cold water enemas, hitting his fingernails or finger joints hard against
a desk, hitting corns on his feet with a stick and repeatedly dipping
his hands into water at extremes of temperature.

## J. Müller

Johannes Müller accepted many of Reil's ideas about the physiology
of the ganglionic nervous system and partially followed Weber in
arguing for pain as overstimulation of the nerves of touch. But he
specifically rejected Reil and Weber's distinction between cenesthesis
and extracorporeal sensation. This rejection was not the decision of
an empiricist neurophysiologist trying to purge his discipline of
Romantic concepts, though Rothschuh[26] depicts Müller in this way.
Rather it was a radical assertion of the equivalence of sensations of
internal and external cause, as expressed in various versions of his
famous doctrine of specific nerve energies. Riese & Arrington[27] have
demonstrated convincingly that the earliest version of the 'doctrine'
was the product of extensive autoexperimentation with subjective
visual phenomena. In the mid-1820s Müller provoked a range of
visual sensations, or phantasms as he called them, by manipulating
his own internal state. For example, he undertook prolonged
exercises of his imagination and even starved himself into a delirious
state. These 'subjective experiments' were grounded in a
post-Kantian interest in the role of the percipiens in perception and

were described in *Über die phantastischen Gesichtserscheinungen* (1826). Müller concluded that man, reaching out for objective reality, reaches only his own sensations: 'Of outer objects we only know of their action on us in terms of our energies'.[28] To put it another way, the sensation provoked by a stimulus depends much more on the nerve than on the stimulus. All that matters about the stimulus is that it be of the right sort to act as a stimulus upon that particular nerve. Thus stimulation of the retina by pressing one's eyeball, or by an object in space, or by the effects of self-starvation all result in an identical sensation. Müller was radically asserting the equivalence of adequacy and effect of internal and extracorporeal stimuli in sensory physiology. This position undercut any distinction between bodily and extracorporeal sensation – or between cenesthesis and touch. Note that the key notion of a 'specific nerve energy', intrinsic to the nerve itself, was a vitalist element in Müller's thought that his pupil Helmholtz challenged strongly.

Before commenting on the relative influence of Reil, Weber and Müllers' ideas on authors after 1846, I want to draw attention to the passages in *Elements of Physiology*[29] that address pain, cenesthesis and the doctrine of specific nerve energies[30]. The following is one clear statement of the doctrine:

> The nerves of the senses are not mere passive conductors [with special susceptibility for certain impressions], but...each peculiar nerve of sense has special powers or qualities which the exciting causes merely render manifest. Sensation, therefore, consists in the communication to the sensorium, not of the quality or state of the external body, but of the condition of the nerves themselves, excited by the external cause. – We do not feel the knife which gives us pain, but the painful state of our nerves.[31]

One might almost say that Müller is arguing here that cenesthesis is the only sensation we have, since any sensation is nothing more than an awareness of the state of the body, specifically its nerves.

In the section on the sense of touch[32] he included pain, pleasure, heat, cold and touch under 'common sensibility' as opposed to the special senses. Whether the stimulus was internal or external was irrelevant. Müller explicitly rejected the Weberian distinction between touch and *Gemeingefühl:* 'Cenesthesis is not a peculiar sense, but merely the common sensibility of the internal parts of the body'.[33] This led to consideration of the unclear sensations emanating from the sympathetic nervous system. He followed Reil on this, arguing that visceral sensations are indistinct and feeble because only the strongest impressions are transmitted through the ganglia, which act as semi-conductors.[34]

The vitalism at play in Müller's writing is exemplified in this extract:

> In inquiring into the nature of the forces resident in the nerves, it is necessary to study the action of all kinds of stimuli upon them...In chemical processes, reagents give rise only to products, combinations, and decompositions; applied to... the nerves, their effects, however various they themselves may be, are never other than manifestations of the proper forces of the bodies acted on...all influences acting on the nerves either excite them, or produce an altered state of their excitability;...the most different causes produce the same effect, because that on which they act possesses but one kind of excitable force, and because agents in themselves the most different act here by virtue of the same quality, that of stimuli.[35]

In this passage Müller seems to doubt whether the phenomena of sensation will ever prove reducible to physics or chemistry. His scepticism about the possibility of measuring the velocity of nervous impulses and Helmholtz's achievement of this within Müller's lifetime are well known.

Müller equivocated about Weber's idea of pain as overstimulation. He certainly did not accept that overstimulation of the retina could give rise to pain – the retina and optic nerve could yield only visual sensation:

> Mechanical irritation of the sensitive nerves of the trunk...produces merely the varieties of common sensation, namely, pain and the sensation of touch; irritation of the retina, on the contrary, gives rise to no pain...but to the perception of light.[36]

He thought, like Weber, that 'The sensation of pain seems to depend on the violence with which the nerves of touch are irritated',[37] but would not extend this to nerves serving other sensory modalities. At another point he argued that overstimulation tends to damage nerves so that no sensation is transmitted thereafter.[38]

### After 1846

Schiller[39] cites a number of other German medical authors of the first quarter of the nineteenth century who followed Reil's thinking on cenesthesis. The writings of Brack, Stierling, Walther and Naumann are unfortunately unavailable in translation. But what of the second half of the century? Did Reil's Romantic concept prevail or did

Müller's hugely influential book (and pupils and journals) render it obsolete? Secondary sources (Boring[40] and Schiller[41]) suggest that pain as cenesthesis found support from Erb (1876), Funke (1880), Blix and Goldscheider (early 1890s). One primary source in which Reil's views on pain as cenesthesis are maintained, despite a clear appreciation of Müller's teachings in other areas, is *The Principles of Medical Psychology* by Ernst von Feuchtersleben.[42] In the first section of what is recognizably a textbook of psychiatry he offers a Reilian physiology.

According to Feuchtersleben, the human begins life with *Ursinn*, an obscure, generalized innate sensation of existence that is prior to any perception at all. Then cenesthesis, based on activity in the ganglionic nervous system, and sense perception, grounded in the cerebrospinal nerves, begin. Pain may arise from the *Ursinn*, cenesthesis or from the sense of touch. Cenesthetic sensations include heaviness, atony, hunger, thirst, sexual stirrings, as well as those pains emanating from the ganglionic nervous system.[43]

A cursory perusal of general histories of psychology or the physiological titles of Helmholtz will confirm that the special senses were more intensively researched in the second half of the nineteenth century than was pain. A comprehensive comparison of the sensory physiology and psychology of perception of Müller and Helmholtz is to be found in Lenoir.[44] It is tempting to digress onto this topic here, but the key point for the argument I am developing is simply that Helmholtz, both in his experimental work and in more general discussions of theory of perception (e.g. *Concerning the perceptions in general*, 1867[45]), concentrated on vision and hearing rather than cutaneous sensation. The most obvious explanation for this is the lack of any known receptor organ for pain prior to von Frey's work of the 1890s. I would like to suggest that an enduring conceptual distinction between cenesthesis and extracorporeal sensation was also a factor contributing to the relative neglect of pain in the new fields of sensory physiology and experimental psychology in the period 1846–1894. In support of this viewpoint I shall describe Wilhelm Erb's comments on pain as *Gemeingefühl* from his influential *Handbuch der Krankheiten der peripheren cerebrospinalen Nerven* of 1874–8.[46]

Erb studied medicine from 1857 to 1861 at Heidelberg University and was Assistant to Professor Friedreich there during the period in which the *Handbuch* was written. He succeeded Friedreich in the chair in 1883[47]. Five pages of the book lay out Erb's position on pain. He begins by explaining that he, like Valentin, Wundt and

Eulenberg, favours the Weberian notion of pain as overstimulation. Pain is a bodily feeling resulting from excitation of any sensory process that exceeds a certain intensity. It 'is that *Gemeingefühl* which is not an expression of a particular quality of sensation but only of a certain degree of that sensation.'[48] He was aware of Fechner's concept of a sensory *limen*, or threshold, but states 'no sharp threshold can be defined where the sensation of pressure or temperature ends and the sensation of pain begins'. Usually it is overstimulation of the nerves of touch that causes pain, but high intensity light or sound (such as detonations) can cause pain through overstimulation of these special senses.

Erb's discussion closes with a very interesting passage on the origin of pathological pain, as opposed to experimental pain. He argues that all pain arises when either stimulus intensity or the excitability of the sensory apparatus increases. He points out that the first of these is rare in pathological pain:

> Only in a few cases are we dealing with an increasing strength of the stimulus and then there are rough mechanical processes involved; in the majority of cases we are forced to assume...alterations in the sensory apparatus which cause an increased excitability in the sensory apparatus.

He calls this hyperaesthesia and says it cannot be explained until molecular or nutritive alterations in the nerves are better understood.

> The main thing still remains the state and reaction of the consciousness itself and that of the central sensory apparatus, whereas the peripheral apparatus and conducting pathways have nothing more to do with pain other than that they receive excitations and conduct them to the centre.

Thus Erb, like Müller, puts the focus on the central nervous system function of the pain patient rather than on the lesion or stimulus.

## 2. Pain Without Lesion and Cenesthesis

We have seen in Chapters One and Two how French and British doctors answered the problem of apparently lesionless pain in terms of distant lesions or an expanded concept of lesion (the invisible, functional lesion) or as an hallucination due to brain disease. In this section it will be shown that two German psychiatrists, Reil and Feuchtersleben, accounted for pain without lesion, both as an isolated symptom and in the context of neuroses (hypochondria/hysteria), in terms of disordered cenesthesis. This was a novel solution that depended on German Romanticism. Weber and Müller's views on pain without lesion and cenesthesis require more cautious characterization. Müller actually saw all sensation as cenesthetic. He was so comfortable with the physiological equivalence of 'subjective' and 'objective' sensations that lesionless pain was no longer problematic for him after the 1820s.

## Reil

Reil's account of disordered cenesthesis has been reconstructed from summaries of 'Hubner's' 1794 thesis in Schiller[49] and Starobinski,[50] *Rhapsodies on the application of the mental cure to mental disturbances* (1803) in Marx[51] and *Das Zerfallen der Einheit des Koerpers im Selbstbewusstsein* (1808) in Harms.[52] In the 1794 thesis, overfunction of cenesthesis is portrayed as the cause of hypochondria, pica, bulimia, polydipsia and nymphomania. The *Rhapsodies* focused on disturbances of consciousness *(Bewusstsein)*, circumspection *(Besonnenheit)* and attention *(Aufmerksamkeit)*. Circumspection was the ability to attend to various internal and external perceptions simultaneously, in a balanced way, while attention was the ability to focus voluntarily on one percept. Disturbance of either could be at play in cases of lesionless pain. According to *Das Zerfallen* cenesthesis can be weakened or destroyed, resulting in a range of disturbances of bodily sensation including left–right disorientation, loss of self-identity, the belief that one is made of glass and liable to shatter, etc. Given the range of symptoms attributed to a deranged *Gemeingefühl*, and that pain was the classic example of bodily sensation, it seems almost certain that Reil explained pain without lesion in these terms. However, the untranslated primary sources would repay further study seeking a fuller picture of the subtle distinctions Reil drew between, for instance, self-consciousness *(Selbstbewusstsein)* and cenesthesis *(Gemeingefühl)*.

## Feuchtersleben

Four decades later, some 15 pages of Feuchtersleben's 1845 monograph were devoted to pathologies of cenesthesis. Exalted cenesthesis draws attention to internal sensations causing pain.[53] For example, when rheumatism 'excites pain suddenly without any perceptible organic alteration' this is explained by 'elevated cenesthesis'[54] Pain at a distance from lesion and phantom limb pain are explained in similar terms:

When pain is felt in quite a different organic region from that in which the cause is situated, this is often an altered cenesthesis, which unfortunately as easily misleads the medical man as the patient. To this...too, we may refer the feeling of pain in the situation of amputated limbs.[55]

For Feuchtersleben, hypochondria and hysteria are 'in essence nothing but a cenesthesis abnormally heightened in all directions'.[56] Symptoms include hyperaesthesia of the vegetative nerves, disordered digestion, self-centredness and 'a contradiction between the subjective complaints of the patient and the objective phenomena in the organs complained of'[57] The proximate cause of hypochondria is the ganglia conducting, rather than blocking, visceral sensation[58] – this is the orthodox Reilian view. Distant causes include heredity, melancholy temperament, chronic bowel disorder, sexual excess and reading medical books. This exalted bodily sensation is more marked in women 'in consequence of the greater delicacy of the nervous system in the female sex'[59] and motor symptoms are more marked in hysteria (women) than in hypochondria (men).

### Weber & Müller

The positions of Weber and Müller in relation to pain without lesion and cenesthesis require cautious elaboration. Weber turned to the symptoms of pain and fatigue in neurotic patients in the closing paragraph of *Der Tastsinn*:

> In patients, particularly hypochondriacs and hysterics, stimuli which might be so weak as to be unnoticed by healthy persons, can cause vivid sensations of common sensibility. Many believe, unjustifiably, that the cause of these phenomena is an exaggerated sensitivity in the nerves. Rather, it would appear that various organic functions in such patients are susceptible to slight stimuli due to various types of abnormality or affliction. Dysfunction then causes a further dysfunction, resulting in pain. In such debilitated persons, moderate exertion of the muscles rapidly brings on fatigue and pain: this is not because the nerves are more excitable, but because the muscle substance is impaired and, after only very brief activity, undergoes changes which result in fatigue and pain.[60]

Thus Weber did not favour a central origin for the pains of neurotics, rather highlighting the debilitated condition of their muscles.

Müller drew a rather sharp distinction between pain at a distance

from lesion, which he called sympathetic pain and attributed to
'radiation' (see Chapter Four below), and pain without lesion. He
discussed the latter at some length in Book 5, volume II of the
*Elements*[61] in a section on the sense of touch. For Müller, pain
without a stimulus was in one sense an impossibility. All sensations
arose from causes, be they internal or external. This is certainly not
to say, as Morris[62] did, that after Müller pain was either 'real' (i.e.
accompanied by an obvious lesion) or else imaginary. Rather, Müller
allowed such a wide variety of causes, including internal and even
mental causes, that pain without lesion was rather unproblematic:

> Sensations dependent on internal causes are in no sense more
> frequent than in the sense of touch...Neuralgic pains...afford striking
> examples of subjective sensations...The mind also has a remarkable
> power of exciting sensations in the nerves of common sensibility; just
> as the thought of the nauseous excites sometimes the sensation of
> nausea, so the idea of pain gives rise to the actual sensation of pain in
> a part predisposed to it...These sensations from internal causes are
> most frequent in persons of excitable nervous systems, such as the
> hypochondriacal and the hysterical, of whom it is usual to say that
> their pains are imaginary. If by this is meant that their pains exist in
> their imagination merely, it is quite incorrect. Pain is never imaginary
> in this sense; but is as truly pain when arising from internal as when
> from external causes; the idea of pain only can be unattended with
> sensation, but of the mere idea no one will complain. Still, it is quite
> certain that the imagination can render pain that already exists more
> intense, and can excite it when there is a disposition to it.[63]

Thus, although pain was always physiological and never
imaginary, mental acts such as memory, attention and imagination
were among the internal physiological causes Müller enumerated. In
short, 'external agencies can give rise to no kind of sensation which
cannot also be produced by internal causes'.[64] Subjective pain was an
hallucination and, Müller emphasized, hallucinations have a vivacity
that sets them quite apart from mere imagination or ideas:

> Phantasms or hallucinations are perceptions of sensations in the
> organs of the senses, dependent on internal causes, and not excited
> by external objects. These phenomena have been repeatedly
> confounded with mere ideas...But the very belief in their reality is
> owing to their being seated in the senses, and having all the
> truthsomeness of real sensations; moreover, this belief in their reality
> is not an essential character of such phenomena.[65]

He develops this last point by contrasting the hallucinations of the insane with the 'visions' that may be induced by manipulating healthy subjects such as himself. Hallucinations of the insane involve loss of insight while in 'visions' insight is maintained while the sensory phenomena remain just as vivid and 'truthsome'. We now express this as a distinction between hallucination and pseudohallucination. At first glance, he thus concurred with the French alienists in regarding pain without lesion as a hallucination. However, in drawing this distinction between hallucination with and without insight he was arguing against the view that hallucinations were only to be found among the insane, as a result of a diseased brain. Rather, he insisted on the physiological equivalence of hallucinated sensations (with preservation of insight) and sensations with external objects. Pain without lesion could thus be explained without invoking insanity.

## Notes

1   There was no such nation as Germany for most of the nineteenth century, rather a number of smaller states. For simplicity of presentation the word Germany will be used anachronistically without inverted commas in this chapter.

2   Boring, 1942, 463–9, *Sensation and Perception in the History of Experimental Psychology.*

3   Merskey & Spear, 1967, *Pain: psychological and psychiatric aspects.*

4   Morris, 1991, *The Culture of Pain.*

5   Cranefield, 1957, *The organic physics of 1847 and the biophysics of today.*

6   Tuchman, 1993, *Helmholtz and the German medical community.*

7   Riese & Arrington, 1963, *The history of J. Müller's doctrine of the specific energies of the senses: original and later versions.*

8   Müller, 1838, *Elements of Physiology.*

9   Boring, 1942, *Sensation and Perception in the History of Experimental Psychology.*

10   Schiller, 1984, *Coenesthesis.*

11   Starobinski, 1990, *A short history of bodily sensation.*

12   Marx, 1990, *German Romantic Psychiatry, Part I.*

13   *Ibid.*

14   Rothschuh, 1973, *History of Physiology.*

15   Risse, 1972, *Kant, Schelling and the early search for a philosophical science of medicine in Germany.*

16   Risse, 1976, *Schelling, 'Naturphilosophie' and John Brown's system of medicine.*

17  Leary, 1982, *Kant, Fichte and Schelling.*
18  Clarke & Jacyna, 1987, *Nineteenth-century Origins of Neuroscientific Concepts.*
19  Marx, 1990, *German Romantic Psychiatry, Part I.*
20  Weber, 1846, *Der Tastsinn und das Gemeingefühl .*
21  *Ibid.*, 151–3.
22  *Ibid.*, 154.
23  *Ibid.*, 225.
24  *Ibid.*, 227.
25  *Ibid.*, 224.
26  Rothschuh, 1957, *History of Physiology.*
27  Riese & Arrington, 1963, *The history of J. Müller's doctrine of the specific energies of the senses: original and later versions.*
28  Müller, 1826, *Uber die phantastischen gesichtserscheinungen.* Quoted in Riese & Arrington, 1963.
29  Müller, 1838, *Elements of Physiology*     .
30  This exercise is limited by the poor quality of the translation of *Elements* into English as described by Clarke & Jacyna (1987) in their bibliographical essay.
31  *Ibid.*, 766.
32  *Ibid.*, 1324–32.
33  *Ibid.*, 1087
34  *Ibid.*, 662.
35  *Ibid.*, 612–13.
36  *Ibid.*, 613.
37  *Ibid.*, 1327.
38  *Ibid.*, 614.
39  Schiller, 1984, *Coenesthesis.*
40  Boring, 1942, *Sensation and Perception in the History of Experimental Psychology.*
41  Schiller 1984, *Coenesthesis.*
42  Feuchtersleben, 1847, *The Principles of Medical Psychology.*
43  *Ibid.*, 83–93.
44  Lenoir, 1993, *The eye as mathematician.*
45  Helmholtz, 1867, *Concerning the perceptions in general.*
46  Erb, 1876, *Handbuch der krankheiten der peripheren cerebrospinalen nerven.*
47  Bryan, 1994, *Wilhelm Erb.*
48  Erb, 1876, 13, *Handbuch der krankheiten der peripheren cerebrospinalen nerven.*
49  Schiller, 1984, *Coenesthesis.*
50  Starobinski, 1990, *A short history of bodily sensation.*

51  Marx, 1990, *German romantic psychiatry, Part I* .

52  Harms, 1960, *J.C.Reil.*

53  Feuchtersleben, 1847, 215, *The Principles of Medical Psychology.*

54  *Ibid.*, 216.

55  *Ibid.*, 218.

56  *Ibid.*, 222.

57  *Ibid.*, 223–4,

58  *Ibid.*, 225.

59  *Ibid.*, 227.

60  Weber, 1846, 253, *Der Tastsinn und das geimeingefühl*

61  Müller, 1838, 1324–32, *Elements of physiology.*

62  Morris, 1991, *The culture of pain.*

63  Müller, 1838, 1331–2, *Elements of physiology.*

64  *Ibid.*, 1059.

65  *Ibid.*, 1392.

# 4

## Reflexion and Depression

## Pain Without Lesion in mid-century German and British 'Neurological' and 'Psychiatric' Writings: 1840–55

### 1. Reflexion, Irradiation and Eccentricity – Müller, Laycock and Romberg

The deceptively simple-looking question 'When did neurology begin?' has attracted some historical attention. *Garrison's History of Neurology*[1] seems content to offer a 40 year period in which the discipline gradually appeared – between Romberg's *Manual* (1840–1846)[2] and Charcot's appointment as a Professor in 1882. Spillane[3] argues that the mid-century writings of Romberg in Germany and Russell Reynolds in England represent an early 'descriptive' neurology rather than the mature 'analytic' discipline of Gowers' *Manual* of 1886–8.[4] Bynum[5] emphasizes that the history of specialization varied from nation to nation. For example, the strong mid-century neuropsychiatric tradition of Griesinger and Meynert in Germany had no equivalent in England. He argues that 'nervous patients' in England were cared for by physicians in the early nineteenth century but the emergence of the mature specialty of neurology in the years 1870–1890 saw patients with nervous disorders lacking structural lesions passed to the care of psychiatrists and others.

Dating the origin of neurology is thus a problematic, and potentially historically sterile, business. I therefore propose to focus upon a small number of individuals who are widely regarded as seminal influences on the emerging discipline and to explore their intellectual influences and influence, concentrating on their writings about pain at a distance from, or without, lesion.

Clarke & Jacyna[6] have brilliantly demonstrated the influence of German Romanticism and Marshall Hall's concept of the reflex on both Müller in Germany and Laycock in England. In fact, the pattern of influence between English and German neurophysiological thought was very complex with Müller citing Laycock approvingly and Müllerian sensory physiology, as encapsulated in Romberg's three laws, directly influencing English physicians such as Handfield-Jones up to three decades later. Thus it is probably defensible to group the mid-century writings of all these actors together.

To summarize a great deal, Marshall Hall was the first to use the term 'reflex arc' to refer to a sensory input to and motor output from the spinal cord. He was adamant that such processes were always unattended by consciousness and automatic and that the brain was not involved. His attempts to account for a number of nervous system disorders in terms of these spinal reflex arcs have been described as 'unsuccessful'[7] though he did build up a large private practice that he handed on directly to Russell Reynolds. Müller took up the notion of reflexion but modified it such that there could, in certain circumstances, be conscious awareness or sensation associated with a reflex, i.e. the brain as well as the cord could be involved.[8] The sensations associated with sneezing, coughing, vomiting and ejaculation, all activities previously regarded as sympathies, could now be explained. In addition, he suggested that spinal irritation was a state of exhaustion and excitability of the central organs of the nervous system caused by excessive excitement of the genitals. In this state minor sensory stimuli cause large reflex motor reactions.[9] Thus both Hall and Müller in the 1830s were striving to account for nervous disorders unaccompanied by lesion using a new physiology of reflexion.

However, it is Müller's sensory physiology that is of more relevance to the topic of pain without lesion. Some of this was covered in Chapter Three above but here I wish to introduce his concept of 'radiation' since it was modelled on reflexion. In a section of the *Elements* entitled 'Of the Radiation of Sensations' he briefly described a clinical phenomenon that was impossible to explain given his new insistence upon the absence of any functional connections between peripheral nerve fibres. How, he asked, do sensations in disease extend to parts not affected? For example, how can the pain of toothache spread to involve the face, then the arm and even fingers on one side? How do these secondary, 'sympathetic' radiations of pain occur?[10] His answer is that the radiation must occur centrally, in the spinal cord or brain. This process is analogous to communication between centripetal sensory and centrifugal motor fibres in reflexion. But in the case of radiation there is spread from one centripetal sensory fibre to many other sensory fibres surrounding it:

> the mere radiation of an impression, from one sensitive nerve in the
> substance of the brain or cord, so as to affect the origins of other

sensitive fibres, will be sufficient to produce sympathetic sensations.[11]

Thus he proposed a mechanism analogous to the reflex arc, but confined entirely to centripetal sensory fibres, to explain pain at a distance from disease. We have already seen in Chapter Three that he also had a clear position on pain without lesion, allowing mental acts such as concentrated attention, memories and acts of imagination as internal physiological stimuli giving rise to sensations identical to those from external stimuli. I shall return to Müllerian physiology again with Romberg's work, but first an extended reading of Thomas Laycock's *Nervous Diseases of Women* from 1840 will be offered to illustrate how Hall and Müller's ideas were taken up in an English context.

Thomas Laycock [1812–1876] was educated at University College London but extended his medical education by studying in Paris (1834) and took his MD at the University of Göttingen in 1839. He was influenced by Marshall Hall and extended the spinal reflex arc to include the brain in the period 1840–1844. He developed this in both *A Treatise on the Nervous Diseases of Women; comprising an inquiry into the nature, causes and treatment of spinal and hysterical disorders*[12] and in his lectures to the British Association for the Advancement of Science of 1844. Jacyna[13] and Clarke & Jacyna[14] have argued that the parallel, largely independent extensions of the reflex concept by Müller and Laycock were both driven to a great extent by the monist philosophy of mind of German Romanticism. Jacyna also portrays the development of a dynamic physiological psychology in mid-century England as an attempt to regain ground lost with the fall of phrenology – depicted by Jacyna as a static 'anatomical psychology'. In my opinion Laycock's 'extension of the doctrine of the reflex functions of the spinal cord to include the encephalic ganglia'[15] has been overemphasized at the expense of his other preoccupations of the early 1840s. In the Preface and Introduction to *Nervous Diseases* the elucidation of 'the action of the will on the sensorial fibres of the brain, the nature and laws of sensation' is portrayed as an equally central aim of the book. A specific clinical problem drives this interest:

> The most common and injurious error is that which confounds the neuralgic form of hysteria with inflammation of some vital structure... Limbs have been amputated when no organic disease has existed... the successful treatment of this class of diseases, more than any other, requires such a combination of general knowledge, sound judgment, and medical tact, as falls to the lot of few who are

91

engaged in the daily hurry and turmoil of general practice.[16]

Thus Laycock pinpoints pain without lesion as a key problem challenging the clinician and demanding in-depth knowledge of the latest sensory physiology. Laycock dwells on physiological explanations for 'hysterical or neuraemic neuralgias' in Chapters 6, 10 and 11 of Part I. He portrays his idea of placing the sensorial fibres under the power of the will as building on Bell, Hall and Müllers' legacy. It was now understood that the pain provoked by irritating any point on a nerve fibre is referred to the peripheral distribution of that nerve. So, from the point of view of consciousness, central and peripheral stimulation of sensitive nerves are indistinguishable. Sensation is a state of the sensitive nerve, not a perception of the quality of an external stimulus. Now, for Laycock, the explanation of hysterical neuralgia is irritation of some part of the sensitive nerve in the brain or spinal cord causing a sensation that is indistinguishable from that caused by inflammation at the peripheral end of the same nerve due to organic disease.[17] But what is the nature of this central irritation? Again following Müller very closely, he regards mental acts as sufficient internal stimuli:

> changes in the sensorial fibres of the encephalon may originate internally as well as externally... it may be hypothetically supposed that there is a surface on which sensorial fibres terminate, connected with ideas, which is analogous to the sensitive fibres on the skin... the action of the will on the sensorial fibres during acts of memory and attention is followed by remarkable phenomena... By an act of will we can excite new sensations. Let an individual concentrate his attention upon the interior of his head for a few minutes, and he will experience various sensations in the skin.[18]

He went on to suggest that such acts of attention are often 'involuntary or instinctive'.[19]

I am arguing that there is a strand in Müller and Laycocks' writings, neglected to date by historians, in which psycho-physiological explanations for pain without lesion were sought. Laycock regarded this endeavour as of equal importance to the extension of the spinal reflex to the brain. Both authors credited mental acts as sufficient internal sensory stimuli and this argues strongly against those who have sought to depict the neurophysiology of the period as a reductionist enterprise that obscured all appreciation of a 'psychology' of pain. For example, Merskey & Spear[20] have portrayed Müllerian sensory physiology as the conceptual base for the discovery of a rigid neural architecture for pain, the pain pathway. Once Schiff and others had traced this pathway in the spinal cord, the argument continues, pains became either real (i.e. due to external organic stimuli) or imaginary and thus appreciation of the phenomenology of pain was lost. It should by now be apparent that I regard this depiction of Müller's thought and influence as profoundly mistaken. The position Müller and Laycock take on lesionless pain was close to the philosophical school of German Idealism, with the emphasis on the subjectivity of the person in pain rather than the 'objective' judgements of a medical observer.

To return to Laycock's text, the difference between the sexes was a crucial given: 'the nervous system of the human female is allowed to be sooner affected by all stimuli, whether corporeal or mental, than that of the male'[21] and 'affectability' was the best word to summarize this difference. The excessive sensitivity of the female was manifested through the nervous system but was rooted in the blood that nourished the nerves. Thus women have less fibrin than men, and hysterical women have depleted blood, especially after menstruation. 'Perhaps a good general term for the whole class of hysteric and hypochondriacal diseases would be Neuraemia'.[22] Hence hysterical and neuraemic neuralgia were one and the same condition.

Laycock devoted two chapters to the topic of laterality of the nervous disorders of women:

> All nervous diseases do not attack the left side in preference to the right... However, of most functional diseases of the nervous system [including hysterical neuralgias] it may be remarked generally, that they are observed to affect the left side rather than the right.[23]

Chapters 7 and 8 of Part III deal with the sensory symptoms of spinal and hysterical disorders in detail. Spinal, sternal, costal, rectal and anal neuralgias are covered, along with pain in the left side and hysterical neuralgias of the head and face that are clinically indistinguishable from true tic douloureux.

Laycock's text is obviously steeped in the new Müllerian physiology but in the *Manual* of Moritz Romberg,[24] published in German in exactly the same period, we find an even clearer summary of those aspects of Müller's thought that were relevant to the neuroses.

Romberg was *Privatdozent* at the University Hospital, Berlin from 1830 until he assumed the Directorship in 1840. Johannes Müller was the Professor of Anatomy and Physiology at the same university from 1833 onwards and greatly influenced this clinician.

Romberg had translated Bell's *The Nervous System of the Human Body*[25] into German and his famous *A Manual of the Nervous Diseases of Man* was published in parts between 1840 and 1846. It went through three editions by 1857 and the second of these was translated into English in 1853.[26] The organization and content of the book were influenced by Bell, Müller and Hall. The division of the neuroses into 'neuroses of sensibility' and 'neuroses of motility' was premised on Bell, the three laws Romberg proposed were a crystallization of Müller's work on sensation and the reflex theory of hysteria includes repeated references to Marshall Hall. Working from the English translation I shall now offer a reading of the large section on 'neuroses of sensibility' to see whether Romberg attended to pain without lesion and, if so, what terminology and theorization he offered.

Neuroses of sensibility arise from a 'vital process by which an abnormal variation in the excitability of the centripetal nerves is produced'.[27] These variations are quantitative, not qualitative, namely an increase or decrease in excitability: hyperaesthesia and anaesthesia respectively. The abnormal excitability may be manifested as 'conscious sensation' or as 'reflex action'. Only the former are relevant to explaining pains. Romberg then specifies the three physiological 'laws' governing sensory nerves:

1. THE LAW OF ISOLATED CONDUCTION – adjoining fibres are not connected in the periphery.
2. THE LAW OF SYMPATHY OR IRRADIATION OF SENSATIONS – 'irritation is propagated from the fibre originally excited to other centripetal nerves'[28] within the central organs of the nervous system.
3. THE LAW OF ECCENTRIC PHENOMENA – 'Every sensation, as it becomes perceptible to consciousness, is referred to the periphery of the sensitive fibre'.

In addition to these Müllerian principles, Romberg states that the type of sensation provoked by a stimulus depends on the type of nerve excited, thus hyperaesthesia of cutaneous nerves causes pain while hyperaesthesia of nerves of special senses causes 'phantasms' (i.e. hallucinations). This restatement of the doctrine of specific nerve energies reiterates the physiological similarity of lesionless pain and other hallucinations. Finally Romberg reminds the reader that the brain is not a passive receptor in sensation. Rather the active percipiens reacts to intensify or even to create sensations de novo, for example through acts of imagination in hypochondriasis.

The hyperaesthesiae share certain nosological features: persistent, uniform symptoms with periodic exacerbations representing no danger to life. These criteria are very similar to the new 'positive' definition of neurosis by Georget published in 1840. López Piñero[29] has emphasized that this redefinition went beyond the 'principle of negative lesion' on which Pinel initially grounded the class of the *névroses*. Such efforts to describe the positive features of the neuroses imply that Romberg and Georget rejected the view that the class of neuroses would gradually shrink away as pathological anatomy uncovered more and more structural lesions to explain these conditions. In fact, as was made clear in the Preface to the second edition of the *Manual*, the whole thrust of Romberg's approach to nervous disorders was against pathological anatomy in favour of the new physiology. The later detailed observations on hysteria made by Charcot and Freud fall within this tradition of defining the distinctive physical and psychopathological features of neuroses rather than dismissing the category as provisional, a mere diagnosis of exclusion. This will be discussed again in the later chapters.

Romberg divided the hyperaesthesiae into two distinct orders, governed by different physiological laws: hyperaesthesiae from irritation of peripheral nerves were shaped by the law of isolated conduction while hyperaesthesiae of central origin were under the sway of irradiation and reflection. Having stated these general principles, Romberg moves on to detailed sections on hyperaesthesiae of cutaneous nerves (neuralgias), special senses (hallucinations), sympathetic tracts, spinal cord and brain (hypochondriasis). Hysteria is not covered under the neuroses of sensiblity since for Romberg it is entirely governed by reflection (rather than irradiation) and its manifestations are automatic, involuntary reflex motor actions (rather than sensations).

Romberg was rather unconcerned about the presence or absence of structural lesions, given that all sensory symptoms represented hyperaesthesia, i.e. pathophysiology. Even when lesions were clearly present it is the dysfunction they provoke, rather than their mere presence, that accounts for the symptom. For this reason Romberg greatly expanded the referent of the term 'neuralgia' to include all pains confined to the distribution of one or more cutaneous nerves, including those arising from obvious injury to the nerve or due to neighbouring tumours etc. Spillane complains of Romberg that 'there is little to suggest that he appreciated the importance of clinico-pathological correlation'.[30] In my opinion this misses an important principle that Romberg was seeking to establish, namely that sensory symptoms were always mediated by dysfunction and never simply attributable to the presence of structural lesion.

Romberg described facial, lumbosacral, cervical and intercostal neuralgias and cited both Swan and Brodie as experts on these conditions. The most detailed case history of facial neuralgia in a 'respected Berlin merchant' aged 57 affords an opportunity to pause to review the state of the art of bedside sensory examination and post mortems in the 1840s.

> During the intervals [between exacerbations of pain] I was occasionally permitted to test the sensibility of the two sides [of the face] with a needle. The result was invariably the same, *viz.* exalted sensibility of the left side of the face in the entire range of the fifth pair [of cranial nerves]. There was no difference of sensibility on the two sides of the tongue; both sides tasted alike and normally.[31]

The post mortem examination was sufficiently detailed to reveal an aneurysm of the carotid artery pressing on the 'Casserian ganglion of the Vth nerve' as the cause of the neuralgia. Incidentally, Romberg regarded this case as an excellent illustration of the law of eccentric phenomena since the irritation was clearly central while the altered sensation was referred to the periphery.

In the discussion of neuralgias of the lumbosacral plexus Romberg raises the importance of making the differential diagnosis between sciatica and Brodie's local hysteria, that is, between neuralgic and hysterical pain. The latter was more often seen in young women, with left-sided symptoms and even accompanied by hysterical fits while true sciatica was evenly distributed across the sexes with no lateralization in the body. Sciatica demanded treatment aimed at removing the cause of irritation where known (e.g. accelerate the labour or relieve constipation) while local hysteria was best tackled through moral treatments, with particular care to divert the attention of the sufferer from the painful part to external interests.[32]

As Shorter[33] and López Piñero[34] have emphasized, Romberg devoted considerable rhetorical energy to attacking the diagnosis of spinal irritation, which he regarded as a peculiarly 'British' error. For Romberg, hyperaesthesiae of the spinal cord could be manifested consciously, as pain, in which case the diagnosis was neuralgia, or unconsciously, as motor symptoms, that is as reflex hysteria.[35]

Hypochondriasis, or Hyperaesthesia Psychica, was defined as 'that frame of mind in which abnormal sensations are excited and maintained by directing the attention to impressions',[36] and more specifically, dwelling on ones own sensations. Indolent professional men were most at risk, especially medical men. The symptoms

96

included fixed pains and the conviction of a localized malady
followed by endless self-examination, reading, medical consultations
and frequent changes of doctor. Romberg distinguished this
condition from melancholia by contrasting the rather grandiose
aspect of the hypochondriacal self-diagnosis with the 'self-negation'
of melancholia. The moral management of hypochondria, he said,
should be aimed at diverting the attention through 'billiards, fencing,
gymnastics, playing a musical instrument... Pedestrian tours, and
sojourning in beautiful mountain scenery, riding, swimming,
driving, sailing, shooting'.[37] Romberg emphasized that reassurance is
quite ineffective and, echoing Müller, that, although the imagination
can initiate sensation, there is no such thing as an imaginary
sensation:

> In perception it makes no difference whether the irritation takes
> place at the central or peripheral termination of the fibre, and
> whether it is induced by directing the attention to it or by a
> mechanical, chemical or organic cause.[38]

I have argued that the writings of both Laycock in England and
Romberg in Germany were influenced by Hall's concept of the reflex
arc, especially as extended by Müller. But of even greater importance
for the specific problem of pain without lesion were the new laws of
sensation that Müller had expounded. In particular the laws of
irradiation and of eccentricity provided physiological explanations
for pain at a distance from lesion while the doctrine of specific nerve
energies, asserting the radical equivalence of internal and external
stimuli, rendered pain without lesion conceivable. As I emphasized
above, these pains were not actually uncaused. Rather, mental acts
such as focusing attention, exercising the imagination and
reminiscence were attributed with causal power as internal stimuli.
Thus what might now be called the phenomenology of pain
perception was fully incorporated in the new neurophysiological
model.

## 2. British Physiological Psychology – Carpenter and Holland

That both Laycock and Romberg were influential within their own
national contexts and beyond is not in doubt. For example, Jacyna[39]
has detailed how the mid-century physiological psychology of
Carpenter and later the thought of Hughlings Jackson were directly
influenced by Laycock. However, the emphasis in this history has
been on the transmission of the extended concept of the reflex so I
thought it important to briefly reexamine Carpenter's 'mental

physiology' from the point of view of pain without lesion. Did he regard it as exactly equivalent to any other hallucination and did he preserve the Müllerian position that hallucinated sensation was physiologically identical to sensation arising from an obvious material cause?

The first edition of *Mental Physiology* was not published until 1876.[40] But it was an expanded version of the sections on psychology in the much earlier fifth edition of the *Principles of Human Physiology* (1855).[41] In exploring Carpenter's adoption of Laycock's ideas it seems prudent to start with this earlier text. In the Introduction to the 1855 monograph Carpenter failed to acknowledge either Laycock or Holland. The most important section for our purposes is a 60-odd page account 'Of the Mind, and its Operations'. He rehearses materialist and spiritualist philosophies of mind, then states that the physiologist cannot help but be acutely aware of mind–body interactions. These instances do not threaten freedom of will or the immaterialism of man's soul for Carpenter. He simply regards it as clear that on occasions mental agency can excite nerve force or nerve force can excite mental energy. Mind cannot influence Matter directly but can do so indirectly, via a 'dynamical metamorphosis' as Force.[42] Thus sensations without external, material referents are unproblematic:

> [in all kinds of sensation] as the change of which the Mind is informed is not the change at the peripheral extremities of the nerves, but the change communicated to the Sensorium, it hence results that external agencies can give rise to no kind of sensation which may not also be produced by internal causes... The various phases of common sensibility often originate thus.[43]

Internal causes of such 'subjective sensations' include inflammation of tissues or 'peculiar conditions of the Encephalon itself', such as the state of dreaming. Thus Carpenter invokes Müllerian physiology in support of sensations without lesions. He also appeals to the notion of irradiation to explain pain at a distance from lesion. Pain is felt in the tip of the penis in a case of bladder stone because

> these impressions [from the bladder pathology] produce sensorial changes, which are referred to their parts, in virtue of some central track of communication with them, analogous to that through which reflex movements are excited.[44]

These are dubbed 'reflex sensations'. On the next page Carpenter mentions the law of eccentric phenomena, so the centrality of the new sensory physiology is quite clear.

Enlarging on the theme of pain without lesion he brings a distinction between internal sensation (cenesthesis) and external sensation into play, citing Reil explicitly on this. Ideas, he suggests, can produce an impression in the nerves of internal sensation. This impression is then referred to the nerves of the external senses and hence is felt as a peripheral pain. The specific case Carpenter seeks to explain here is that of a butcher who impaled his arm on a meat hook. He was in agony until it became clear, some time later, that only the sleeve of his coat had been torn.[45] On the following page, Carpenter echoes the Reilian model of the human infant developing from a cenesthetic creature into a being capable of linking external objects to internal sensory experiences – that is to say, capable of interpreting sensations, capable of perception. At other points in this large text Carpenter seems reluctant to place pain as either an internal or external sensation. Pleasure and pain are described as 'simple feelings' that are close to aesthetic or moral or emotional sensibility. Pain may be associated with either ideas or sensations.[46]

In a chapter on 'Sensibility in General and the Sense of Touch' E.H. Weber is repeatedly cited but no account of pain sensation is presented to match the rather detailed discussion of touch. And when the bodily sensations (common sensibility, cenesthesis) are listed, pain is omitted: hunger, thirst, nausea, sexual senses and the 'sinking stomach' of intense emotion are the only examples. These apparent inconsistencies are eliminated in the *Principles of Mental Physiology* of 1876[47] where it is made clear that Carpenter follows Weber in viewing pain as overstimulation of any sensory apparatus, but lacking an anatomy of its own.[48] In this text he goes on to make an explicit link between localized bodily pain and generalized feelings of malaise or depression, both being mediated by cenesthesis.[49]

Carpenter's main influence, apart from Laycock, was the man to whom he dedicated his *Mental Physiology* of 1876 – Henry Holland. I shall briefly explore a few passages in Holland's *Chapters on Mental Physiology*[50] to provide another example of how pain without lesion was handled in mid-century British physiological psychology. Chapter 3 on the 'Effects of Mental Attention on Bodily Organs' is most relevant to our theme. It was first written in 1839, Holland explains, under the influence of Müller's idea that attention can augment the intensity of ordinary sensations. 'Attention' means directing or fixing consciousness on a part of the body. This may be volitional but is more often due to attention being drawn to a region by impressions. A third way in which attention can be focused is under the influence of certain mental states, such as hysteria or mesmeric trance. In these latter states 'past images and memories rise up unbidden to perplex both sensations and acts by mingling with them'.[51] In hypochondria 'the patient, in fixing his consciousness with morbid intentness on different organs, creates not merely disordered sensations, but often, also, disordered actions in them'.[52] Attention may be directed to internal organs, specific sensory modalities or to the brain itself. Interestingly Holland mentions that attention tends to focus upon 'a region, or compound member of the body, [rather] than upon a particular organ or texture [= tissue]'.[53] This predates the comments of Russell Reynolds and Charcot (see Chapters Five & Six below) on the spatial distribution of ideogenic sensations by over two decades. Holland is uncertain of the physiological mechanism behind these phenomena stating only that 'the nerves are in some manner excited by the act of attention' and referring the reader to Carpenter. What is striking to me here is the influence of Reilian physiology, with its subtle distinctions between attention (*Aufmerksamkeit*), circumspection (*Besonnenheit*) and self-consciousness (*Selbsbewusstsein*)[54] via Müller, on this British author. A considerable Victorian literature on 'morbid introspection' ensued which has been very well surveyed by Clark.[55] I hope this brief glance at Holland's text is sufficient to raise the possibility that this British genre of medical writing had its roots in German Romanticism.

I shall now turn from mid-century British physiological psychology to German 'psychiatry' to continue my exploration of the influence of the new sensory physiology.

### 3. Pain Without Lesion as Mental Depression – Griesinger

I now consider a monograph that, according to Marx[56] and Micale[57] was probably the most influential psychiatric textbook of the century: Griesinger's *Mental Pathology and Therapeutics*, first published in German in 1845, i.e. contemporaneously with Romberg's *Manual*. The second edition, of 1861, was the version that became internationally renowned, and the English translation was published in 1867.[58] Although Griesinger eventually became Professor of Psychiatry in Berlin in 1865, the book was first written when he was at Winnenthal in the 1840s. Book 1 is devoted to general considerations. Griesinger asserts that mental diseases are brain diseases and that the lesions range from 'simple irritations without perceptible changes of structure' to obvious hyperaemias, inflammation, etc.[59] The new clinical method, premised on clinico-pathological correlation is unfortunately not yet applicable to mental diseases:

> Cerebral pathology is, even in the present day, to a great extent in the same state which the pathology of the thoracic organs was in before the days of Laennec. Instead of proceeding in every case from the changes of structure of the organ, and being able to deduce in an exact manner the production of the symptoms from the changes in the tissue, it has very often to deal with symptoms of which it can scarcely give an approximation to the seat, and of whose mode of origin it is totally ignorant.[60]

He makes a number of 'Preliminary Physio-pathological Observations on Mental Phenomena'. 'The brain is an immense reflex apparatus'[61] in which intelligence (including perception) represents an intermediate field between sensory input and motor output. Griesinger drew a distinction between sensation and perception. The former was always based in irritation of a sensory nerve while the latter may or may not be:

> A great number of other perceptions are not immediately provoked by irritation of the sensitive nerves, but are produced internally by the functions of the brain, which are independent of all sensorial excitation. When intelligence excites sensation the result is illusion and hallucination.[62]

Both sensation and perception are subject to the law of eccentric phenomena and referred to the periphery[63] and subject to the doctrine of specific nerve energies, with a radical equivalence between external and internal stimuli:

> the energy special [to a given sensory nerve] can be put into play not only by their normal external irritants, but also by internal irritation... in particular... by morbid irritation [of the brain].[64]

Thus Griesinger follows Müller closely on all these matters.

He states that perceptions can be painful in two ways: as localized bodily pains or as 'a state of general uneasiness, of bodily malaise, without localized pain'. Local pains are typical of hypochondriasis while the non-localized pain is central to the diagnosis of melancholia.[65] Both modes of painful perception are preoccupying and tend to diminish all other perceptions. 'Elevation of the I' weakens external impressions and 'a hypochodriacal subjectiveness and egotism' is induced.[66] As localized physical pain reduces muscular activity so non-localized mental pain diminishes volition.[67] Clearly Griesinger regarded physical and mental pain as closely related. For him, the issue of localization distinguishes them rather than any dualist consideration. Chronic localized bodily pain without lesion and the mental pain of melancholia are both 'states of mental depression'. The former is hypochondriasis while the latter is melancholia proper. I will confine myself to hypochondriasis, but only after underlining once again the monism inherent in Griesinger's physiology.

In 1818 Heinroth[68] had excluded 'diseases of the senses', such as hysteria and hypochondria, from the category of insanity because they entailed no permanent loss of reason, only hallucination. In contrast, Griesinger, while agreeing that hallucination alone was insufficient to clinch a diagnosis of insanity, argued that 'The hypochondriacal states represent the mildest, most moderate form of insanity'.[69] For him it was a *folie raisonnante mélancholique* in which the 'strong feeling of BODILY illness' [capitals in the original], together with depressed mood, gave rise to false opinions without global intellectual derangement.[70]

> All the parts of the sensory nervous system may be the seat of morbid
> sensations, often very painful (… as if his head would burst – as if
> he were empty, dead, pierced, torn in pieces, etc.).[71]

The false beliefs of suffering serious disease then arise as 'attempts at explanation' and are expressed 'in the most graphic and ludicrous language'.[72] A series of case histories, taken by Griesinger from other authors, illustrate these points.

Case 1.[73] Mademoiselle H., a 21 year old. Lost her usual cheerfulness and secluded herself for a year. All her thoughts were concentrated on continuous pain in the right hip. Physical examination was normal. The patient later expressed the belief that her guts were about to spill out through her abdominal wall.

Case 2.[74] Mr M-. Married at 31, hepatitis at 32. Afterwards 'everything was a perpetual source of pain and annoyance to him'. He had constant pain in the right hypochondrium that he ascribed to the liver, fearing cancer. The conviction waxed and waned, being stirred up by incidental bouts of fever affecting the mucous membranes. The pain sometimes shifted position, e.g. to right shoulder tip, lumbar region, bladder and urethra. He gave up work and died three years later due to complications of investigations of the bladder at the hands of a lithotritist whose opinion he had sought.

In addition to this picture of hypochondriasis, Griesinger also makes further comments on hallucinations and on the relationship between bodily pain and insanity. Hallucinations are 'intra-cerebral phenomena' and may occur in any sensory modality. While Griesinger follows Esquirol in distinguishing between hallucination (percept without object) and illusion (misperception of an object) he points out that 'In the skin, and in the viscera, hallucinations and illusions cannot be distinguished from each other'.[75] I would add that this is one important way in which pain without lesion constitutes a special problem compared to, say, auditory illusions and hallucinations.

To summarize, Müllerian sensory physiology is to the fore once again in this text. In addition, Griesinger places the phenomenon of pain without lesion at the centre of the 'states of mental depression'. When manifested as local bodily pain the diagnosis is hypochondriasis and when non-localized suffering is prominent melancholia is present. This monism is explicable given Griesinger's temporal and geographical proximity to German Romanticism. Just as Müller is depicted by some historians as the founder of a reductionist neurophysiology, so Griesinger is usually remembered as a materialist or somaticist. In my opinion both of these caricatures neglect the monist legacy of Romanticism that is evident in their writings on pain. Marx[76] has rightly emphasized that the materialism at play in Griesinger's early work was very different from that to be found in Meynert and other later 'somaticist' German psychiatrists.

At this point it is worth pausing to reprise and carefully distinguish three somewhat distinct solutions to the problem of pain without lesion I have found at play in mid-century German and English writings. For Reil, Feuchtersleben and Carpenter the crucial distinction is between bodily sensation (cenesthesia) and extracorporeal sensation. Pain without lesion is regarded as a phenomenon of abnormal cenesthesia. Pain with lesion is explained in terms of the overstimulation of any extracorporeal sensory modality. For Müller, Romberg, Laycock and Holland all sensation is cenesthetic. Pain without lesion is seen as the result of internal physiological stimuli, including attention, memory, imagination and emotion. For Griesinger all pain is cenesthetic; when localized it is felt as bodily pain, when unlocalized it is experienced as mental pain or melancholia. This bald summary is a caricature which obscures the profound similarities between these authors.

## 4. Dualism, Localization and British Neurology

I want to close this section by examining a text written by Russell

Reynolds in 1855 because it illustrates how the importance of localization, at the expense of subjective experience, was reasserted as the new German neurophysiology was taken up in British proto-neurology. To put this another way, this text can be read as the superimposition of empiricist pathological anatomy on Romantic neurophysiology. The result, I shall argue, was the loss of monism and the beginnings of a dualist discipline.

John Russell Reynolds was educated at University College London and was awarded an MD in 1852. He moved into Marshall Hall's old house in London and took over his entire private practice of 'nervous' patients in a manner which attracted criticism from within the medical profession at the time. His 1855 monograph *The Diagnosis of Diseases of the Brain, Spinal Cord, Nerves & their Appendages*[77] was written in the context of working with the same clinical population that had supported Hall's exposition of the reflex arc. Later Russell Reynolds went on to greater things, becoming Professor of Medicine at University College London in 1865, Physician to the Queen in 1878 and President of the Royal College of Physicians from 1893–5.

The part of the book I wish to dwell upon is the opening chapter entitled 'The Objects [i.e.Aims] of Diagnosis, and its limits' and Appendix B 'On the relation between functional changes and structural lesions'. It is my contention that these very clear expositions of the relation between symptom and lesion unite the physiological neurology of Romberg and more traditional pathological anatomy. The conclusion is an affirmation of the importance of precise localization in clinical medicine, while the exact nature of what it is that has been so precisely pinpointed remains as problematic as ever. In my opinion this passion for localization, regardless of the precise pathology to be found in that place, defined the new discipline of neurology. On the opening page Reynolds enumerates the three aims of diagnosis in nervous diseases:
1. 'given the symptoms to discover the locality of lesion'
2. 'Given the symptoms and the organ affected, to find the nature of the affection', by which he meant specifically the functional disturbance or 'dynamic affection'
3. Determine the exact nature of the structural lesion or 'anatomical/static/organic condition'.

Expanding these aims he states that the differential between diseases intrinsic and extrinsic to the nervous system is a key point in localization.[78] Functional disturbances may be divided into acute and chronic, febrile and afebrile and increased or decreased function.

Neuralgias, hallucinations and hypochondria all point to excessive function while anaesthesiae suggests diminution of function.[79] Structural lesions need not be present at all: 'it is not unphilosophical to believe in the existence of morbid functions without demonstrable physical lesion'.[80] Thus Reynolds supports the distinction between functional and structural diseases of the nervous system, giving hysteria, neuralgia and epilepsy as examples of the former.

Appendix B offers a more detailed insight into Reynolds' position. He begins by stating that although the class of dynamic/functional/inorganic nervous diseases – the neuroses – has been 'diminished' by the discovery of more and more 'correspondent physical changes in the organs', many remain as apparently 'purely dynamic derangements'.[81] The conclusion Reynolds reaches is that 'there are functional derangements which no anatomical lesions can explain'. Furthermore, even when structural lesions are found in nervous disorders

> the mechanical changes, such as haemorrhage, congestion, softening, etc., do not cause the symptoms directly, but by the intervention of secondarily induced alterations in the minute organic processes.[82]

I would suggest that Reynolds' interest in the problem of the neuroses (symptoms without structural lesions) was grounded in his clinical work with Hall's private patients. The emphasis on the mediation of dysfunction between obvious structural lesion and symptom implies a marriage of Rombergian physiological thinking with pathological anatomy.

The 1860s saw the appearance of monographs devoted to functional nervous disorders in contrast to the neurology of structural lesions. It is to these that I now turn in further pursuit of writings about pain without lesion. The appearance of this sharp distinction, premised upon the presence or absence of structural lesion, reflects the reassertion of empiricism, and specifically pathological anatomy, as Romberg's new discipline was taken up in an Anglo-French context. Instead of starting from the phenomenology of perception, as Müller did, and trying to leave room for subjectivity, the active percipiens, in neurophysiology, Briquet, Brown-Séquard, Charcot, Gowers and others reduced the patient to their symptoms and visible signs, that is, to a perceptum of the medical gaze. In order to achieve this they had to play down inter-individual variation in symptoms and signs of neurosis. What was at stake was not the primacy of the nomothetic over the idiographic but the exclusion of a whole range of lived experiences from the field of neurology proper.

## Notes

1 McHenry, 1969, *Garrison's history of neurology.*
2 Romberg, 1853, *A manual of the nervous diseases of man,* second edition.
3 Spillane, 1981, *The doctrine of the nerves: chapters in the history of neurology.*
4 Gowers, 1886, *A manual of diseases of the nervous system.*
5 Bynum, 1985, *The nervous patient in eighteenth- and nineteenth-century Britain: the psychiatric origins of British neurology.*
6 Clarke & Jacyna, 1987, 114–47, *Nineteenth-century origins of neuroscientific concepts.*
7 *Ibid.*
8 *Ibid.,* 124–5.
9 Muller, 1838, 710–11, *Elements of physiology.*
10 *Ibid.,* 697.
11 *Ibid.,* 699.
12 Laycock, 1840, *A treatise on the nervous diseases of women; comprising an inquiry into the nature, causes and treatment of spinal and hysterical disorders.*
13 Jacyna, 1982, *Somatic theories of mind and the interests of medicine in Britain.*
14 Clarke & Jacyna, 1987, *Nineteenth-century origins of neuroscientific concepts*
15 Laycock, 1840, ix, *A treatise on the nervous diseases of women.*
16 *Ibid.,* 2.
17 *Ibid.,* 99–100.
18 *Ibid.,* 109–10.
19 *Ibid.,* 111–12.
20 Merskey & Spear, 1967, *Pain: psychological and psychiatric aspects.*
21 Laycock, 1840, 76, *A treatise on the nervous diseases of women.*
22 *Ibid.,* 84.
23 *Ibid.,* 202.
24 Romberg, 1853, *A manual of the nervous diseases of man,* second edition.
25 Bell, 1836, *The nervous system of the human body.*
26 Romberg, 1853, *A manual of the nervous diseases of man.*
27 *Ibid.,* 1.
28 *Ibid.,* 2.
29 López Piñero, 1983, *Historical origins of the concept of neurosis.*

30   Spillane, 1981, 288–9, *The doctrine of the nerves: chapters in the history of neurology.*
31   Romberg, 1853, 38, *A manual of the nervous diseases of man.*
32   *Ibid.*, 59–69.
33   Shorter, 1992, *From paralysis to fatigue: a history of psychosomatic illness in the modern era.*
34   López Piñero, 1983, *Historical origins of the concept of neurosis.*
35   Romberg, 1853, 152–55, *A manual of the nervous diseases of man,* second edition.
36   *Ibid.*, 178.
37   *Ibid.*, 187.
38   *Ibid.*, 186.
39   Jacyna, 1982, *Somatic theories of mind and the interests of medicine in Britain.*
40   Carpenter, 1876, *Principles of mental physiology.*
41   Carpenter, 1855, *Principles of human physiology.*
42   *Ibid.*, 553.
43   *Ibid.*, 562.
44   *Ibid.*, 563.
45   *Ibid.*, 565–66.
46   *Ibid.*, 666.
47   Carpenter, 1876, *Principles of mental physiology.*
48   *Ibid.*, 171–2.
49   *Ibid.*, 173–5.
50   Holland, 1858, *Chapters on mental physiology.*
51   *Ibid.*, 96.
52   *Ibid.*, 104.
53   *Ibid.*, 82.
54   Marx, 1990, 362, *German romantic psychiatry, Part 1.*
55   Clark, 1988, *Morbid introspection, unsoundness of mind and British psychological medicine.*
56   Marx, 1970, *Nineteenth-century medical psychology: theoretical problems in the work of Griesinger, Meynert and Wernicke.*
57   Micale, 1990b, *Charcot and the idea of hysteria in the male.*
58   Griesinger, 1867, *Mental pathology and therapeutics.*
59   *Ibid.*, 7.
60   *Ibid.*, 8.
61   *Ibid.*, 24.
62   *Ibid.*, 28.
63   *Ibid.*, 30.
64   *Ibid.*, 33.
65   *Ibid.*, 34.

66   *Ibid.*, 35–6.

67   *Ibid.*, 37.

68   Heinroth, 1818, *Textbook of disturbances of mental life.*

69   Griesinger, 1867, 211, *Mental pathology and therapeutics.*

70   *Ibid.*

71   *Ibid.*, 212.

72   *Ibid.*, 213.

73   *Ibid.*, 217–18.

74   *Ibid.*, 218–19.

75   *Ibid.*, 102.

76   Marx, 1970, *Nineteenth-century medical psychology: theoretical problems in the work of Griesinger, Meynert and Wernicke.*

77   Russell Reynolds, 1855, *The diagnosis of diseases of the brain, spinal cord, nerves & their appendages.*

78   *Ibid.*, 2–6.

79   *Ibid.*, 6–9.

80   *Ibid.*, 10.

81   *Ibid.*, 240.

82   *Ibid.*, 244.

# 5

## Functional Nervous Disorders in French and British Medical Texts: 1859–1871

The clear distinction between structural and functional diseases of the nervous system that Russell Reynolds made in the mid-1850s has been described. The preeminent importance of localizing a lesion – be it structural or functional – to the developing discipline of neurology has been noted. Now, before turning to primary sources on functional nervous disorders, I want to pause to review one question. What was the referent of the term 'functional' in French and British medical thought in the 1850s?

I have argued, after López Piñero,[1] that the speculative functionalism of Broussais and his followers, notably the concept of irritation, was seized upon at first as an invisible process that served as an explanation for the lesionless symptoms of neurosis. Its temporal aspect was largely ignored in the literature on spinal irritation, for example. In the 1830s and 1840s Hall, Müller and Romberg began to describe some laws of nervous system function and dysfunction. These laws set limits on the scope of speculation about the nature and location of dysfunction underlying symptoms such as pain without lesion. In this chapter I shall try to show how further laws of this sort were added in the 1860s, notably decussation and inhibition. These new laws added further specificity to the term 'functional'.

Perhaps an even more important body of work at the mid-century rendered functional lesions visible and quantifiable at the laboratory bench for the first time. Lesch[2] and Rey[3] have drawn attention to Bernard's animal experiments with atropine, strychnine and curare in the 1850s, which he saw as a chemical or functional dissection of the body. For example, curare 'destroys movement but remains without effect on sensation'. Henceforth 'functional nervous disorders', the neuroses, had new reality. As Canguilhem put it:

> Claude Bernard, unlike Broussais... supported his general principle
> of pathology with verifiable arguments, protocols of experiments
> and above all methods for quantifying physiological concepts...
> From here on we know exactly what is meant when it is claimed that

disease is the exaggerated or diminished expression of a normal function.[4]

### 1. Briquet on Pain in Hysteria

Although Bernard, and others in the *Société de Biologie,* denounced nomothetic clinical research in favour of crucial experiments with single animal preparations, news of their findings might have given hope to clinicians struggling with the neuroses. And we need not look far to find one such doctor. Many of Bernard's human subjects in the decade 1844 to 1854 were supplied by Rayer at the Charité hospital.[5] Pierre Briquet, a Paris-trained physician, arrived at the Charité in 1846 and began collecting data on hysteric inpatients. Thus, during the period in which Briquet's *Traité clinique et thérapeutique de l'Hystérie*[6] was conceived and written, the meaning of the term 'functional nervous disorders' was being redefined on the doorstep. No doubt Briquet and Bernard would have had their differences over methodology. As Mai & Merskey[7] have emphasized, Briquet's *Traité* was an early venture into what is now known as psychiatric epidemiology – descriptive data on 430 cases seen in the decade 1846–1856 constituting the bulk of this monograph. Bernard argued against such statistical exercises throughout his career. Nonetheless, it is conceivable that awareness of Bernard's research helped Briquet to approach hysteria as a disease with as many regularities in its presentation and causation as any other. He made his position clear in the Introduction: *'pour moi l'hystérie est une névrose de l'encephale'.*[8] It was this aspect of the book that so impressed Charcot.

In my close reading of Briquet's *Traité* I will highlight material on pain without lesion. The descriptive data supported two old observations on the symptomatology of hysteria and identified three aetiological factors that were continuously taken up by others until the 1890s.

The old observations that Briquet confirmed were the preeminence of sensory symptoms, especially pain, in hysterical patients and the left-sided predominance of these symptoms. For him, the principal and pathognomonic symptom of hysteria was extreme sensibility of the nervous system and pains.[9] In Part II of the book, on symptomatology, he lists very many 'algias' without structural tissue changes. The mild form of hyperaesthesia was an exaggerration of normal feeling from the part while in the more severe form spontaneous pains were felt. Any part of the body was at risk, though *myosalgie, céphalalgie* and *rachialgie* (backache) were most common. Other pains included *dermatalgie, epigastralgie, pleuralgie, coelialgie, thoracalgie* and *arthralgie*. Briquet commented that true neuralgia, or *névralgie ordinaire*, was rare in hysteria. His explanation is most revealing of his view of the pathology of hysteria. He argued that, since hysteria was a disorder of the affective areas of the brain and since peripheral nerves were merely simple conductors, peripheral nerve function was undisturbed in hysterics.[10] The ubiquity of muscle pain in hysterics was explained as owing to the passions finding their expression in the muscles. Oft-repeated passions pushed the muscles from a physiological to a pathological state. This was typically seen in patients chronically exposed to sad moral affections.[11] The distinction between such *myosalgie hystérique* and chronic muscular rheumatism hinged on the left-sided preference of hysterical pain.[12]

The issue of laterality of sensory symptoms runs through the entire text. For example, he observed that *rachialgie* was five times more common on the left than on the right. Harrington[13] has considered Briquet's views on lateralization in detail. It is clear from her research, which draws on his remarks about Broca's new work in the *Bulletin de L'Academie Imperiale de Médecine* of 1864–5, as well as the *Traité*, that Briquet was opposed to an explanation of unilateral hysterical pains based on cerebral assymetry. He thought that dysfunction of the emotional and sensory areas of the brain was at play in hysteria but, following Bichat's 'law of symmetry', argued that these areas were bilaterally represented. His preferred explanation for the left-sided predominance of pains was more fatiguable muscles on the left side of the body.[14] By 1874 Brown-Séquard had explained the clinical phenomenon quantified by Briquet in terms of cerebral assymetry. In *Dual Character of the Brain* he wrote: 'the right side of the brain serves chiefly the emotional and hysterical manifestations'.[15] Luys at the Charité also favoured a centre for emotion in the right hemisphere as the explanation for a range of hemi-hypnotic phenomena in 1881 (see Chapter Six below).

Briquet divided the discussion of aetiology traditionally, into predisposing and proximate causes. But his use of data collected systematically from 430 patients, and in particular his comparison of the forbears and descendents of hysterical patients with those of normal controls, was rather novel. Georget had found that a good deal of nervous disorder was reported among the parents of hysterics at the Salpêtrière. But Briquet's comparison of the relatives of 354 hysterics with those of 167 healthy women proved the importance of heredity as a predisposing aetiological factor to his own satisfaction.[16] It is not by chance that we find the issue of heredity coming to attention in a French text on a neurosis in the late 1850s. As Dowbiggin has described: 'The 1850s witnessed the emergence of heredity as a focal point of interest in the elucidation of mental and nervous pathology'.[17] The patterns of inheritance envisaged by Morel and Moreau de Tours included transformational heredity and the accumulation of a taint over successive generations of a neuropathic family. Thus the observations of Georget and Briquet lumped together diverse nervous disorders, including epilepsy, deafness, blindness, hypochondria and hysteria, as evidence of degeneracy in these families.[18]

The other predisposing cause Briquet focused on was the sexual life of the patient. A number of competing agendas were at play for Briquet in this area. First and foremost he wanted to demolish the view that hysteria had its roots in the uterus. The fact that this neurosis was 20 times more commonly seen in women than men he attributed to the *mode de sensibilité* of women's brains rather than the possession of a womb.[19] That one fifth of cases had an onset in childhood spoke against the uterine theory too.[20] The second idea he challenged, attributed to Louyer Villermay, was that sexual continence or frustration led to a build up of female genital secretions and hence hysteria. Widows, who Briquet assumed to be sexually abstinent, were not overrepresented in Briquet's population[21] and teenage girls, an age group in which hysteria was common and whom others assumed to be sexually abstinent, were sexually active according to Briquet (68 of the 184 teenage girls in his study were having sexual intercourse).[22] Briquet decided it was sexual activity, especially non-orgasmic excitation of the female genitals, rather than abstinence, that predisposed to hysteria.

It is clear from the *Traité* that Briquet, as well as making the assumptions above, took a very close interest in the past and present sexual lives of his female patients at the Charité. He openly commented on masturbation among inpatients[23] – a topic that remained taboo in hospitals until very recently. He performed extraordinarily detailed examinations of genital sensation in many cases, sometimes repeating this procedure at intervals during a long admission. For example, Marie Gaudin, a 25-year-old, was examined in detail on admission in 1854, and again in 1856. The response to touch and pinprick of right and left nipples, internal and external labia, as well as vaginal sensation and clitoral sensibility in the erect and non-erect state were meticulously documented.[24] In view of this barrage of frankness it seems very odd that Charcot accused Briquet of prudery, thus:

> The work is an excellent one, the result of minute observation and patient industry, but it has perhaps one weak side; all that relates to the ovary and the uterus is treated in a spirit which seems very singular in a physician. It exhibits a kind of prudery, an unaccountable sentimentality.[25]

Charcot, in public, stripped hysteria of any sexual aetiology while still confessing privately to medical men that *'C'est toujours la chose génitale... toujours... toujours'* according to Freud's later recollections.[26] It thus seems likely that the prudery, if any, was on Charcot's part. Micale[27] has argued that the 'programmatic asexualism' in both Briquet and Charcots' writings was 'a calculated response to ancient but still influential aetiologies of the disease' aiming to 'bring it within the orbit of sober positivist science'. My own view is that Briquet's work was not asexual by any means and that there were elements of sexual hypocrisy and prudery in Charcot's approach.

One interesting question is to ask how Briquet could report so candidly on this material in the 1850s while in the early 1880s Breuer fled an hysterical patient in terror on sensing her attraction to him and possibly his to her? I wonder if the answer lies in the social class of the hysterics concerned and the setting in which they were seen. The Charité inpatients would generally have been poor and uneducated, and thus lent themselves to reduction to objects of nomothetic medical research. In contrast, Anna O. was a well-educated private patient from the same social stratum as Breuer and thus less readily perceived as just one more case. Finally it is possible that the hospital environment in itself protected Briquet from accusations of impropriety while Breuer, working intensively in the patient's home, was more exposed.

In listing the proximate causes of hysteria in order of frequency Briquet formally demonstrated what many earlier authors had mentioned in passing: that emotional upsets or psychic traumas were common. Abuse of children by parents and of wives by husbands was the most frequent cause. Other triggers included fright (for example of witnessing a suicide, fire, crime or battle), annoyances (such as an interfering mother-in-law), stress of migration (say from the country to Paris to go into domestic service) and financial loss. In Chapter Six I shall be claiming that the London surgeon Erichsen inscribed mechanical trauma into the concept of neurosis in the 1860s. Here is an earlier example of trauma being written into a neurosis. But in this case it is a psychological trauma rather than a mechanical trauma. By the time Page, in 1883,[28] insisted that the trauma of railway accidents was psychic rather than corporeal he was merely echoing what some physicians with experience of functional nervous disorders had known for over 20 years.

To summarize, Briquet placed most lesionless pain in women squarely in the category of hysteria, a neurosis of the brain. Indeed certain forms of pain were pathognomonic of hysteria for him. He attributed the precisely localized pain of true neuralgia to dysfunction of peripheral nerves but most headaches, backaches, abdominal and joint pains lacking structural pathology were explained as brain dysfunction.

Micale[29] has pointed out that Briquet's *Traité* was rather less influential than certain other French views of hysteria in the 1860s and 1870s, and that it was only after Charcot drew attention to the work that it became historically significant. For example, Piorry and Négrier developed Romberg's idea of 'reflex hysteria' in the late 1850s, stating that ovarian irritation led to pelvic neuralgia and, by reflex action, to hysteria. Shorter[30] strongly supports this point of view. Both historians emphasize that the notion that genital irritation lay behind hysterical symptoms was the rationale for ovariotomies in these decades.

## 2. Brown-Séquard

Charles Eduard Brown-Séquard was in Paris throughout the 1840s and was instrumental, with Bernard and others, in founding the *Société de Biologie* in 1848. Thereafter, as Aminoff's excellent biography[31] makes clear, mood swings drove him to move repeatedly between London, Paris, Dublin, Mauritius and the United States for the rest of his life. In 1858 he delivered a famous series of lectures to the Royal College of Surgeons in London and two years later requested a post as one of the founder physicians at the hospital in Queen Square, London that is now known as the National Hospital for Nervous Diseases. In the period 1860–63 he was probably Britain's foremost specialist in nervous disorders and developed a busy private practice. After he abruptly abandoned all this in 1863 he had to wait 15 years for his next prestigious appointment. He took over the chair in Medicine at the *Collège de France* in 1878 when Bernard died.

Brown-Séquard is important in the story of pain without lesion for a number of reasons. First, and most famously, he demonstrated the decussation of the sensory conducting tracts in the spinal cord as well as dispatching the erroneous opinion that the posterior columns of the cord white matter conveyed pain sensation to the brain. This research earns him a place in the standard histories of nineteenth-century pain physiology.[32, 33] Whether he, Schiff or Gowers was clearest about the anatomical distribution of sensory pathways in the spinal cord has generated some historical interest. The 'discovery of pain pathways' has been portrayed as a breakthrough[34, 35] and as a disaster.[36, 37] It improved clinicians' understanding of the spatial relationship between pain and pathology but only at the price, according to Merskey & Spear, of reducing a complex subjective experience to a fixed anatomical substrate. Beyond this, little has been said about his ideas on neuroses. Secondly he popularized the concept of inhibition in neurophysiology, as emphasized by Smith.[38] On sectioning the cervical sympathetic nerve of animals he, like Claude Bernard in the 1850s,[39] found that secretions and sensibility were increased in the head, implying that the sympathetic nerve was exercising a tonic inhibitory effect in health. He did not use the word 'inhibition' to describe this phenomenon until the late-1870s, but, as we shall see, the concept was expounded as early as his 1858 lectures to the Royal College of Surgeons.

Decussation and inhibition were thus added to the list of laws of nervous system function that physicians drew upon in the clinic; earlier examples had included the Bell–Magendie law, Müller's laws of isolated conduction, eccentricity, reflexion and irradiation and the doctrine of specific nerve energies. In this way Brown-Séquard's work altered the referent of the term 'functional'. He transformed it in at least one other equally important way too. The nerve sectioning and nerve irritating experiments that he and Bernard performed independently provide a good example of how 'functional lesions' became increasingly demonstrable, and therefore believable. Bernard's curare experiments have already been mentioned in this respect. I will present some material from just two of his numerous publications. First the classic lectures to the Royal College of Surgeons in 1858 in which decussation and inhibition were discussed, then a monograph on functional nervous affections from 1868 which affords a close look at Brown-Séquard's use of the term 'functional'.

The 1860 monograph *Course of lectures on the physiology and pathology of the central nervous system* delivered at the Royal College of Surgeons of England in May 1858[40] is a much-expanded version of those lectures, with many experiments and case histories added.

Lecture II attacked Longet's idea that the posterior columns of the spinal cord 'convey sensitive impressions to the brain'.[41] Apparently Longet continued to champion this early idea of Bells long after its originator had abandoned it. He criticized Longet for confining his experiments to excitation of nerves and cord rather than sectioning or lesioning as he favoured. Brown-Séquard pointed out that conducting sensation was a completely different functional property than detecting stimuli ('impressionability'). Sectioning the posterior columns caused hyperaesthesia, not the anaesthesia predicted by Longet's view. Lecture III discussed decussation and a series of experiments were summarized to show that 'the conductors of sensitive impressions make their decussation in the neighbourhood of the place of insertion of the sensitive nerves, or roots of nerves, in the cerebro-spinal axis'.[42] This was a novel finding with great clinical relevance. In Lecture IV it was argued that the senses of touch, pain and temperature are anatomically distinct within the spinal cord. In Lecture V many clinical cases of hyperaesthesia were collated from various authors in support of Brown-Séquard's ideas. The histories and findings on examination in life in some of these cases were undistinguishable from Briquet's hysterics. Only the post mortem findings, together with the growing understanding of the functional anatomy of the spinal cord, set them apart. For example Case 13 was a 47-year-old woman admitted to the Salpêtrière in 1855. Numbness and formication in her arms, worse on the left, had begun 3 years ago after 'a violent emotion'. There was mild weakness and loss of the sense of touch in the left hand and violent pains in the left arm, spine and chest. At post mortem examination, after she had died 'of diarrhoea', the whole length of the posterior column of the spinal cord looked yellow and abnormal and was then examined microscopically. This case provides an example of how the developing field of neurology was shrinking the category of hysteria by way of its ever more impressive clinico-pathological correlations.

Experimental work demonstrating the inhibitory effect of the sympathetic nerve was presented in Lecture IX. Sectioning the cervical sympathetic caused increased secretions and sensibility in the animal's head, while galvanizing it decreased these functions. On page 173 there is talk of 'two modes of action of the nervous system' but he did not use the word 'inhibition' until many years later.

Turning to *Lectures on the diagnosis and treatment of functional nervous affections,* what, if anything, did Brown-Séquard have to say about pain without structural lesion? Two alterations of function of sensory conducting fibres could give rise to hyperaesthesia or 'morbid sensations' – increased and perverted powers.[43] These states were seen as the result of irritation of centripetal nerve fibres. Such irritation could be caused by an obvious structural lesion or not. Neuralgia was the term he used for one such irritation in the absence of lesion. Irritation of a given peripheral nerve could produce a great variety of reflex or irradiated effects. For example, infraorbital neuralgia could cause changes in the pupil, the muscles of the orbit or photophobia. Neuralgia, an irritation of a peripheral nerve, could increase or pervert the power of the sensory fibres in the cord leading to further distant pains arising through irradiation or muscular phenomena through reflexion. 'Functional affections' thus had a precise referent in Brown-Séquard's text: symptoms arising at a distance from irritation specifically by processes of irradiation or reflexion. The advance on Broussais's speculative functionalism lay in the new understanding of nervous system function interposed between irritation and distant symptom, an understanding that could be supported with animal experiments.

There is a notable absence of all reference to the mind in these two texts. Unlike many of the authors discussed earlier in this thesis, he did not speculate about the interplay between mind and body in cases of lesionless pain. His thought embraced individual differences between nervous patients but accounted for this in terms of physiological differences. He believed the relative excitability of the parts of the nervous systems varied from one neurotic to the next, rather than placing idiosyncrasy in the realm of mental subjectivity. This supports my depiction of the new discipline of neurology as an enterprise premised on dualism and excluding 'the mental'.

### 3. Russell Reynolds on Ideal Pain

One year after Brown-Séquard's book on functional nervous disorders was published a short paper appeared in the British Medical Journal of 1869 by John Russell Reynolds, by now Professor of Medicine at University College London. After 15 years further experience of nervous disorders since writing his 1855 monograph[44] (see Chapter Four above) he had come to a remarkable conclusion that potentially dented the scope of the discipline of neurology that Brown-Séquard and himself, among others, were so actively developing. He had come to realize that not all clinical presentations of nervous disorder could be explained in terms of localizable neurophysiological dysfunction. In some patients the pattern of symptoms was determined by the patients ideas, emotions, or both, rather than irritation of their nerves. He singled out pain, spasms and paralyses as symptoms that he had seen generated in this manner, entitling his paper 'Remarks on paralysis, and other disorders of motion and sensation, dependent on idea'. This paper has been singled out as the first clear statement of ideogenesis, or more precisely, the pathoplastic role of ideas in the production of bodily symptoms.[45] Ideogenesis means the process by which somatic symptoms are born of ideas rather than caused by diseases.

The novelty of Russell Reynolds' contribution was the emphasis he placed on chronic symptoms arising from ideas. Examples of the immediate effects of strong belief or emotion were widely known, such as the story about the butcher's sleeve and the meat hook in Carpenter's book. But in this paper a number of cases of chronic symptoms shaped by the patient's long term concerns were presented. For example, the chronic pains of a nine year old boy were explained as 'imaginary' or 'ideal'. This was not to say that the pain was not real. The patient suffered. But the pain was portrayed as a persistent hallucinatory after-image of an earlier painful and worrying organic disease, analogous to visual after-images. Note here that the 'reality' of pain was first assured by reference only to the subjective experience of the patient, while a few lines later the 'reality judgment' rests with the doctor, who can identify an 'ideal' pain when he encounters one.

Reynolds explained why hallucinated pain presented the patient with special problems of judgement. In the case of visual after-images there is the possibility of 'confronting the romance of one sense with the realism of another' and so establishing insight into the hallucination

> But in the matter of pain...there is no such correction to be obtained...the physician may find facts enough to guide his mind on the interpretation of the phenomena, but the patient cannot separate the unreal from the real, and is often aided in exaggerating the importance of the former by the kind but ill-advised solicitude of anxious relatives.

Russell Reynolds listed a number of observations that pointed to the 'inorganic' nature of the boy's symptoms: no spinal tenderness, an inability to stand or walk despite a full range of leg movements lying flat in bed, no pain on knocking the soles of his feet when horizontal but great pain on touching the feet lightly on the floor while being held vertical by the armpits. Even his facial expression when complaining of pain was not quite right: 'the expression of countenance is one rather of alarm or fear than of actual suffering'.

I do not know how this paper was received at Queen Square, or elsewhere in Britain, but in Paris Charcot recognized its interest and later cited it in his 'Friday lectures' of the early 1880s (see Chapter Six). Charcot went on to develop a psychophysiological model of ideogenesis in which the patient's ideas were supposed to provoke and shape a localized functional or dynamic lesion of the nervous system (see his discussion of case of Porcz). But, in 1869, Russell Reynolds set ideogenic symptoms in opposition to those caused by a localizable lesion. By adopting this stance Russell Reynolds could not explain ideogenic somatic symptoms neurophysiologically. He did not place them in the field of psychiatry either, emphasizing that in the main such patients with chronic 'ideal' pains or paralyses showed no sign whatsoever of insanity.

I said earlier that this paper 'potentially dented the scope of the discipline of neurology'. In fact it seems clear that both Russell Reynolds and Charcot saw the clinical skills involved in discriminating between ideogenic and neurogenic symptoms as being at the heart of the new specialty. The difference was that while Russell Reynolds thought ideogenic symptoms could be detected and morally managed but not explained by neurologists, Charcot offered a psychophysiological theory that rescued ideogenesis from the metaphysical realm of mind–body dualism.

Does this paper by Russell Reynolds represent the moment when the meaning of the term 'functional' shifted from a physiological to its current psychological connotation? I think the answer is a resounding no. The phrase 'functional nervous disorders' continued to be used to denote neurophysiological dysfunction without structural pathology until the mid-1880s. It only acquired an equivocal meaning after Charcot's work. The purely psychological referent of the word is a twentieth-century phenomenon. These remarks will be supported more fully by the texts examined in the rest of this chapter.

### 4. Handfield-Jones on Functional Nervous Disorders

Bynum has drawn attention to Charles Handfield-Jones's *Studies on Functional Nervous Disorders* as a comprehensive illustration of how this class of disorders were viewed in London around 1870.[46] In an introductory section, on 'some well-established points in neurophysiology and pathology', Handfield-Jones added eleven more laws to the three that Romberg had popularised (ie. isolated conduction, irradiation/reflexion and eccentricity). Among these additional principles available to the late-nineteenth-century nerve doctor were irritation of centripetal nerves and inhibitory influences (from Brown-Séquard), comments on the natural opposition between fever and neuralgia, and parallels between peripheral and central nervous disorders. The example he gave of the latter was alternating pain and melancholic insanity in one patient.[47] Thus making a diagnosis of 'functional disorder' was, by now, much more than an admission of defeat, more than a diagnosis of exclusion.

The comments on the 'natural opposition' between fever and neuralgia illustrate the enduring importance of the temporal pattern, or periodicity, of nervous disorders. This exemplifies Foucault's argument[48] that fevers and neuroses were considered together from Broussais's work onwards.

Having laid out these general principles Handfield-Jones surveyed a large number of conditions. I have singled out only those diagnoses that included pains: headache, spinal irritation, hysteria, hypochondriasis and neuralgias. He divided headache into those varieties where dysfunction was seated in the brain and those where it was seated in the nerves of the head.[49] 'Nervous' headache was due to debilitation and anaemia of the brain and its associated symptom was slowing and dulling of mentation. Its opposite was 'hyperaemic' headache in which congestion of the brain with blood resulted in hypersensitivity of the special senses and restlessness accompanying the pain. 'Sympathetic' headache depended upon irritation in a distant place, typically the gut. The three types of headache due to dysfunction of the nerves of the head were 'neuralgic', 'rheumatic' and syphilitic. Handfield-Jones described one of his cases as 'a good example of neurotic headache'. Case 6, a woman, L.R., aged 44 was married with no children and 'very intellectual'. In childhood she had suffered convulsive hysteria overtreated with leeches applied to the groins. She had been anaemic with headaches ever since. On examination both her facial expression and physical condition attracted comment: 'Has a peculiar expression of suffering and depression, brows rather knit...Slight build...Feeble pulse..'

The passage on spinal irritation[50] steered a middle way between Teale's advocacy and Romberg's outright rejection of the diagnosis. Handfield-Jones left the questions open. Should the term be seen as referring to patients with generalized neuroses, such as hysterics, who happen to display spinal tenderness, or is there a hyperaemic functional lesion localized in some part of the spinal cord? Although the spinal irritation literature had peaked in England around 1840 it is clear that at least some physicians were still considering it seriously 30 years later. Shorter has argued that it remained a popular concept in the spa resorts and Alpine clinics of Europe until as late as 1930.[51] The case histories reveal more details of how Handfield-Jones examined 'spine' patients and his views on the aetiology of chronic neurotic pains. Light and firm pressure, pinching of folds of skin in the lumbar regions, sending a current of air over the skin of the back and the use of compasses to test skin sensibility were all mentioned. The left and right sides of the back were compared using each of these stimuli in turn. As for the cause of such pain, he blames the patients' mothers:

> Sufferers of this class deserve sincere commiseration, though we cannot help smiling at some of their miseries. Their malady is a fearfully real one, no less than insanity...to which it is allied. Mothers who, by foolish fondness, train their children to ways of which such is the ending, are in sober truth guilty of grievous cruelty. Better let a child run all sorts of risks than become a miserable hyperaesthetic.[52]

Here we see a mixture of moral and physical possible causes being put up to explain lesionless pain. This same causal brew was more carefully considered in the passage on hysteria.[53] Handfield-Jones proposed three aetiological routes: constitutional weakness of will, psychic trauma and nerve dysfunction. The first route leads to dissumulation and deceit – these women are basically malingerers and deserve no sympathy. The doctor should make a judgement about when this point is reached and

> Once this limit is passed, and we feel that the patient is no longer trustworthy, we ought to suspend medicine, for otherwise we become, as Mr Carter tells us, most helpful accomplices in her impostures.[54]

Psychic trauma may be chronic – 'poor girls employed as milliners and sempstresses, toiling on...year after year, with almost everything to dispirit and depress them'.[55] – or acute. He mentions the case of a physician who suffered hysterical seizures after spending several hours weeping over his granddaughter's coffin.[56] The nerve dysfunction may be secondary to such psychic trauma or of bodily origin – toxins, exhaustion, reflex irritation.

Pain only figures prominently in three of the thirteen cases of hysteria he presents. Case 7, a 28 year old single woman, had been ill for four years with left-sided head pains and flexion contracture of the left knee. Her cousin, probably her fiancé, had died two months before the symptoms began.

Pain certainly figured in the diagnosis of hypochondria, defined as the presence in the patient's consciousness of some uneasy or distressing sensation, associated often with an apprehension of the existence of some malady with which he has somehow managed to get superficially acquainted.[57]

The symptoms were seen as more constant over time than in hysteria and there were no seizures. A typical sufferer was Mrs C., aged 37, three years into an unconsummated marriage. She complained of lack of sexual desire, pain in the breast, between the shoulders and in the left side of the abdomen. She believed that she was dying of a gynaecological malignancy and was not amenable to persuasion on this matter. She demanded repeated gynaecological examinations that were always normal:

> she questioned me again and again to know if there was not some
> mortal disease, replying to my decided negatives with the demand
> why she suffered such pains if there was no structural lesion.[58]

Such cases, he concluded, were close to melancholic insanity when the beliefs reach delusional proportions. Note here the attention to the patients incessant questioning. Her mental state and speech were being scrutinized along with her physical state and we shall see this was a trend in the later neurological writings of the century (e.g. Allbutt, Gowers).

The passage on neuralgia reveals a wide use of the term. But this neurotic condition was much more fully described by Anstie one year later so his is the account I have chosen to examine.

## 5. Anstie on Neuralgia

Alam and Merskey[59] have traced the expansion and contraction of the referent of the term 'neuralgia' over the course of the nineteenth century. They observe that its meaning expanded between 1840 and 1880, then contracted to the limited meaning it retains to the present. In a nutshell they argue that the original referent was lesionless pain of a certain quality confined to the distribution of a peripheral nerve. In the years between 1840 and 1880 the meaning widened to include a large range of pains, including abdominal pains (visceral neuralgias), cancer pain, pain of obvious peripheral nerve injury as well as pain arising after psychic traumas. They do not offer a very satisfying explanation for this expansion or its sudden reversal in the 1880s. My view is that it was Romberg's attitude to the neuroses that explains the widening of meaning in the 1840s. As we have seen, he saw nerve dysfunction as the cause of all nervous symptoms, so relegating the importance of the presence or absence of structural lesions in, or impinging on, the nervous system. This emphasis on physiology over pathological anatomy allowed him to advocate a very wide use of the term neuralgia to include pains both with and without lesion. The much narrower use of the word in the 1880s and beyond probably owed a great deal to the influence of Gowers' *Manual*,[60] in which he insisted that neuralgia be reserved to denominate pain over the course of a peripheral nerve without 'primary organic lesion'. He used the term 'neuritis' when there was identifiable pathology.

The purpose of this brief digression is to place Anstie's book of 1871 on *Neuralgia and the diseases that resemble it*[61] in relation to these trends. We shall see that he employed a very broad use of the term that included both the pain of cancer and pain of emotional origin as well as the more classical superficial pains. One could go so far as to say that this text represents the climax of the very inclusive use of the word.

Anstie was a physician and medical journalist based at Westminster Hospital from 1860 onwards. He had been taught by Todd at King's College Hospital in the 1850s and was involved in editing both the *Lancet* and *The Practitioner* until his premature death at 41. His monograph on neuralgia was his most famous publication. He introduced the work by arguing that pain is not an hyperaesthesia of the nerves of touch. His main evidence that pain and touch must be mediated by different fibres was a phenomenon which has been repeatedly replicated in cases of neurogenic pain since:

> in parts which are acutely painful a marked bluntness of the tactile perceptions can be detected. The tactile perceptions are, no doubt, conveyed by an independent set of fibres from those which convey the sense of pain.[62]

Thus he argues against Weber's overstimulation hypothesis of pain and in favour of a special pathway for it. The influence of Brown-Séquard may have been at play in this. In addition he regarded pain as a consequence of a 'perturbation of nerve force' in the sense of a 'lowering of function'. He went on to contrast the localizing value of the nerves of common sense (i.e. touch) with the poor guide to the position of pathology that is pain:

> the indications given by pain are vague and untrustworthy, and often seriously misleading... Especially is this the case in the neuralgias, for

more commonly than not the apparent seat of the pain is widely removed from the actual seat of the mischief which causes it.[63]

He defined neuralgia as

a disease of the nervous system, manifesting itself by pains which, in the great majority of cases, are unilateral, and which appear to follow accurately the course of particular nerves, and ramify...into the terminal branches of these nerves.[64]

It was of sudden onset, 'at first unattended with any local change', intermittent and the patient was generally anaemic or otherwise debilitated. Pain from the pressure of extraneural tumours, pain in the aftermath of psychic shock, pain from partially or completely divided nerves, trigeminal neuralgia, mastalgia, visceral neuralgias and sciatica were all included. The pathology was in the central, not peripheral, nervous system in every case:

the essential seat of every true neuralgia is the posterior root of the spinal nerve in which the pain is felt...and...the essential condition of the tissue of that nerve root is atrophy, which is usually non-inflammatory in origin.[65]

Anstie admitted he had no post mortem evidence for this at all. Instead he listed a series of indirect arguments in favour of a central origin. First, neuralgia was a hereditary neurosis. For example it often alternated with another neurosis in a single patient over time. Secondly the pain was clearly influenced, or caused, by emotion, especially 'long-continued mental habit':

Perhaps the maximum of damage that can be inflicted through the mind upon the sensory nervous centres is effected when, to the kind of self-consciousness that is generated by an excessive spiritual introspection there is added the incessant toil of a life spent in sedentary brain work, and chequered with many anxieties, and many griefs which strike through the affections. Doubtless such a combination of morbid mental influences is sufficient of itself to generate the neuralgic disposition in its severest forms, without any hereditary neurotic influence, and without any other peripheral irritations.[66]

Thirdly, he claimed that his model could explain the spread of neuralgic pains from the distribution of one spinal nerve to others through central radiation of irritation.[67]

Anstie's views on the aetiology and pathology of neuralgia are interesting as they draw together several lines of thought that we have already encountered. There is the concept of morbid introspection, the notion of ideas or emotions provoking somatic symptoms as emphasized by Russell Reynolds, the choice of the posterior root established by the Bell–Magendie law, the invocation of Müllerian irradiation and the discussion of hereditary neuroses citing Morel and Moreau de Tours.

The later chapters of the monograph were devoted to the differential diagnosis of neuralgic pain. The most interesting of these concerns the comparison with the pains of hypochondriasis. These were boring or burning rather than the acute, darting pain of neuralgia. The influence of mental attention was described as 'overwhelming' in hypochondria. For example, the hypochondriac may become pain-free when suitably distracted. This was not seen in neuralgia.

## Summary

A number of significant conceptual developments relevant to the problem of pain without lesion occurred in this first decade or so after the formal distinction between structural and functional nervous disorders had been made. Briquet made a good case for the view that lesionless pain, especially left-sided pain, was the most prevalent symptom of hysteria. He went so far as to call it pathognomonic. All three of the aetiological factors he favoured were widely accepted in the four decades that followed: psychic trauma, heredity and the sexual life of the patient. The first two of these reappeared almost immediately in British texts on functional nervous disorders by Handfield-Jones and Anstie.

Brown-Séquard's experiments on decussation and inhibition added two more important principles of neurophysiology that gave substance to the much vaguer notion of 'functional' disorder that had prevailed in the early decades of the century. More significantly, the demonstration of functional lesions in the laboratory by Bernard and Brown-Séquard transformed the meaning of the term 'neurosis' as well as putting meat on the bones of speculative functionalism. Rather than a Pinelian diagnosis of exclusion, 'symptom without lesion', clinicians were now stating the positive presence of dysfunction when they diagnosed neurosis.

Ideodynamism received its first mainstream attention through the paper by Russell Reynolds. Neurologists now needed to attend to the distinction between ideogenic and neurogenic pains. In fact, the differential diagnosis of lesionless pain was beginning to crystallize.

In the writings of Handfield-Jones and Anstie we see at least three varieties of chronic pain without lesion teased apart. The pain of hypochondria or hysteria was clinically quite different from that of neuralgia and this built on Brodie's seminal work. But a third cause of complaints of intractable non-anatomical pain was now mentioned: the hypochondriacal delusions of those suffering melancholic insanity. Here the emphasis was on the verbal complaint rather than the sensory experience of the patient. This underlined the increasing necessity for clinicians to examine the mental state as well as the physical signs of the pain patient and we shall see that trend continued in later writings.

## Notes

1. López Piñero, 1983, *Historical origins of the concept of neurosis.*
2. Lesch, 1984, *Science and medicine in France: the emergence of experimental physiology.*
3. Rey, 1993, 155–6, *History of pain.*
4. Canguilhem, 1989, 75, *The normal and the pathological.*
5. Lesch, 1984, *Science and medicine in France: the emergence of experimental physiology.*
6. Briquet, 1859, *Traité clinique et thérapeutique de l'hystérie.*
7. Mai & Merskey, 1980, *Briquet's Treatise on Hysteria.*
8. Briquet, 1859, 3, *Traité clinique et thérapeutique de l'hystérie.*
9. *Ibid.*, 5–6.
10. *Ibid.*, 245.
11. *Ibid.*, 206–10.
12. *Ibid.*, 212.
13. Harrington, 1987, *Medicine, mind and the double brain.*
14. *Ibid.*, 55–6 & 82.
15. Harrington, 1987, 82, *Medicine, mind and the double brain.*
16. Briquet, 1859, 81–90, *Traité clinique et thérapeutique de l'hystérie.*
17. Dowbiggin, 1985, 191, *Degeneration and hereditarianism in French mental medicine 1840–90.*
18. Briquet, 1859, 81, *Traité clinique et thérapeutique de l'hystérie.*
19. *Ibid.*, 51.
20. *Ibid.*, 73–5.
21. *Ibid.*, 133.
22. *Ibid.*, 75–77.
23. *Ibid.*, 138.
24. *Ibid.*, 57–60.
25. Charcot, 1877, 247, *Lectures on the diseases of the nervous system.*
26. Freud, 1914. Quoted in Noel Evans, 1991.

27. Micale, 1990b, 391–393, *Charcot and the idea of hysteria in the male.*
28. Page, 1883, *Injuries of the spine and spinal cord......*
29. Micale, 1990b, *Charcot and the idea of hysteria in the male.*
30. Shorter, 1992, ch 3 & 4, *From paralysis to fatigue: a history of psychosomatic illness in the modern era.*
31. Aminoff, 1993, *Brown-Séquard: a visionary of science.*
32. Keele, 1957, 112–6, *Anatomies of pain.*
33. Rey, 1993, 223–33, *History of pain.*
34. Keele, 1957, *Anatomies of pain.*
35. Rey, 1993, *History of pain.*
36. Merskey & Spear, 1967, *Pain: psychological and psychiatric aspects.*
37. Morris, 1991, *The culture of pain.*
38. Smith, 1992, 132, *Inhibition: history and meaning in the sciences of mind and brain.*
39. *Ibid.*, 89.
40. Brown-Séquard, 1860, *Courses of lectures on the physiology and pathology of the central nervous system.*
41. *Ibid.*, 11.
42. *Ibid.*, 30.
43. Brown-Séquard, 1868, 12, *Lectures on the diagnosis and treatment of functional nervous affections.*
44. Russell Reynolds, 1855, *The diagnosis of diseases of the brain.*
45. Merskey, 1979, *The analysis of hysteria.*
46. Bynum, 1985, *The nervous patient in eighteenth- and nineteenth-century Britain.*
47. Handfield Jones, 1870, 56, *Studies on functional nervous disorders.*
48. Foucault, 1973, ch 10, *The birth of the clinic: an archaeology of medical perception.*
49. Handfield-Jones, 1870, 416–37, *Studies on functional nervous disorders.*
50. *Ibid.*, 457–67.
51. Shorter, 1992, 38, *From paralysis to fatigue: a history of psychosomatic illness in the modern era.*
52. Handfield-Jones, 1870, 467, *Studies on functional nervous disorders.*
53. *Ibid.*, 468–86.
54. *Ibid.*, 479.
55. *Ibid.*, 469.
56. *Ibid.*
57. *Ibid.*, 487.
58. *Ibid.*, 488.
59. Alam & Merskey, 1994, *What's in a name? The cycle of change in the meaning of neuralgia.*

60. Gowers, 1886, *A Manual of diseases of the nervous system.*
61. Anstie, 1871, *Neuralgia and the diseases that resemble it.*
62. *Ibid.*, 3.
63. *Ibid.*, 3–4.
64. *Ibid.*, 7.
65. *Ibid.*, 110.
66. *Ibid.*, 125.
67. *Ibid.*, 145–7.

# 6

## Functional Nervous Disorders in French and British Medical Writings: 1866–1886

### 1. Trauma and Railway Spine

Trauma was inscribed into the concept of neurosis by surgeons and physicians, notably Erichsen, Page and Charcot, rather than 'psychiatrists'. The impetus for this innovation was the demands of the medico-legal industry that developed in parallel with the rapid expansion in railway traffic. I shall show how Erichsen introduced the importance of a 'shock' to the body while Page clarified that it was the psychic trauma of an accident that was pathogenic.

As Professor of Surgery at University College London in 1866 John Erichsen published six lectures on chronic symptoms, notably paralysis and pain, arising from apparently trivial injuries sustained in railway accidents. An enlarged edition of this work was published in 1882 as *On Concussion of the Spine, Nervous Shock and other obscure injuries of the nervous system*[1] and it is this better known text that I shall describe. Erichsen disliked the apellation 'railway spine' because identical clinical pictures arose from other sorts of civil accidents. He only chose to emphasize railway accidents because of

> the great frequency of their occurrence, consequent on the extension of railway traffic, and because they are so frequently the cause of litigation. There is also a special and painful interest attaching to them from the distressing character of the symptoms presented by the sufferers.[2]

As Trimble [3] has pointed out, over six thousand miles of railway lines had been built between 1836 and 1852 and the railway companies were wealthy organizations, attracting large claims for damages on an unprecedented scale. Erichsen's lectures added fuel to this medico-legal fire because he claimed that many of those disabled after accidents were suffering chronic disease of the spinal cord as a direct consequence of the incident. The precise nature of this disease of the cord was unclear, but disease there was. Erichsen drew upon a medical literature dating from the 1820s in support of an analogy between concussion after head injury and concussion of the spine.

129

He acknowledged that the spinal cord was 'without serious lesion'[4] in such cases but argued that 'molecular changes in its structure' must be present. The 'must' in this view reflected the primacy of the tradition of pathological anatomy which demanded some structural lesion to account for symptoms. Erichsen's voice was therefore typical of the surgical mainstream of his day (cf. Hilton). The novelty was the unusual extent to which he was prepared to speculate about pathology in the absence of post mortem evidence. He suggested a range of pathologies that might lie at the root of the symptoms, including softening and inflammatory changes (such as myelitis or chronic meningitis) and further proposed that these were the consequence of chronic anaemia of the cord.[5]

Erichsen gathered over 50 cases to support his views. Case 27[6] is of particular interest as it concerned a 43-year-old surgeon who was described as active, stout and healthy until being thrown forward in a railway collision some four months prior to consulting Erichsen. He had suffered pain and difficulty walking since the accident. 'He complained chiefly of the spine. He suffered constant pain in the lower part of it...He compared the sensation to that of a wedge or plug of wood driven into the spinal canal.' There was pain and weakness of the right leg as well as loss of 'sexual desire and power'. The patient remained in the same state 12 years later and had been forced to abandon his career 'not owing to any mental incapacity but entirely owing to his bodily infirmities'.

Case 2 [7] provides one further example of the symptom complex Erichsen sought to explain under the rubric of 'spinal concussion'. A 30-year-old painter fell 30 feet to the ground from a ladder. There was no head injury. Ten months later

> He described himself as being languid, depressed, as if going out of his mind. His memory had become very bad...His thoughts were confused...He said he was 'not the same man that he was'...He was never free from an aching, throbbing pain in the back...the [mid-dorsal] spine was very tender on pressure, and the tenderness extended to some distance on either side of it, more especially on the left...

He shuffled with the aid of a stick. Over two years later 'he was still suffering from very severe pain at the lower part of the spine and in the dorsal region' and in fact he never fully recovered. Erichsen concluded that there must have been a 'serious organic lesion' of the spinal cord in this case but was quite unable to specify its nature.

Erichsen was not alone in the 1860s in his ideas about spinal concussion. Hilton predated and shared these concerns, emphasizing the need for rest in cases of 'concussion of the spinal marrow' after railway collisions.[8] Meanwhile Skey found the new compensation industry unacceptable on both medical and legal grounds and felt that the courts would do well to confine compensation exclusively to those with demonstrable structural lesions (Real disease):

> One of such cases I will give you as an example: A man without property or profession brought an action against a railway company for injury to his spine. This statement, on the face of it, is an absurdity. How can a man without property bring an action in law? Well, he applies to a lawyer, who undertakes the case on his behalf, with a certain...understanding as to the question of future payment! Thus the lawyer becomes the plaintiff, and the plaintiff the witness in his own case. The man's injury was made out to the entire satisfaction of the jury, and very heavy damages were awarded by them, coupled with severe comments on the negligence of the railway directors.[9]

He goes on to say that within days of the trial the plaintiff was seen racing another man at walking.

But by far the most celebrated opposition to Erichsen's notion of spinal concussion came in the early 1880s, after his retirement and coincident with the publication of the expanded edition of his 1866 lectures. Herbert Page, a young surgeon at St Mary's Hospital, won the Boylston Prize (awarded by Harvard University) in 1881 for an essay entitled 'Injuries to the Back, without apparent Mechanical Lesion, in their Surgical and Medico-legal Aspects'. This was expanded into book form two years later as *Injuries of the spine and spinal cord without apparent mechanical lesion, and nervous shock....*[10] The opening chapter was devoted to a lengthy review of the pre-Erichsenian literature on spinal concussion, notably the writings of Bell, Abercrombie and Brodie. Page argued that it was almost impossible to injure the spinal cord without significant damage to the spinal column since the cord is so well protected. He also challenged the arguments from analogy with concussion after head injury. In the second chapter he attacked Erichsen directly. He noted that the terms 'spine' and 'concussion' were hopelessly vague and critiqued several of Erichsen's case histories in considerable detail. For example, he objected to Erichsen's Case 2 (see above) on the grounds that many of the symptoms could not possibly be explained in terms of a putative spinal lesion. Yet symptoms of depression, confusion and poor memory were, Page agreed, rather typical of 'railway spine patients'. Page took particular exception to the speculations about myelitis and meningitis. If such pathologies were present after railway injuries, and given that such accidents had by now affected literally thousands of people, why, he asked, was no post mortem evidence available?[11] In the third and fourth chapters Page outlined the symptoms he felt characterized 'railway spine'. The paralysis was, in truth, a 'pseudo-paralysis',[12] a fear of moving because of muscular pains. Back pain and tenderness of the spine on percussion were not indicative of grave spinal cord pathology, rather the reverse.[13] But perhaps the most obvious symptom after railway accidents, according to Page, was 'nervous shock'. This was a generic term for sleeplessness, palpitation and flushing, headache, giddiness on standing, melancholy, hopelessness, noise intolerance, excessive sweating, fatiguable vision and poor concentration (usually described by patients as 'loss of memory').[14] This nervous shock was seen as analogous to the shock associated with, say, loss of blood. Its mechanism was 'a reflex inhibition...affecting all the functions of the nervous system, and not limited to the heart and vessels only'.[15] Here we see two technical terms invoked to explain the puzzling symptom complex associated with lesionless pain – 'reflex' and 'inhibition'. The former term was not that new and has already been examined in my research; however the latter term was very new, being introduced into the field of nervous disorders by Brown-Séquard in the late 1860s (see Chapter Five above). This further supports the suggestion that symptoms without lesion, and perhaps pain above all, drove medical authors to improvise at the limits of current medical theory time and again throughout the century.

For Page, nervous shock could have psychical and corporeal causes but the former were dominant in all railway accidents:

> The incidents indeed of almost every railway collision are quite sufficient – even if no bodily injury be inflicted – to produce a very serious effect upon the mind, and to be the means of bringing about a state of collapse from fright, and from fright only.[16]

While 'the collapse from severe bodily injury is coincident with the injury itself...when the shock is produced by purely mental causes the manifestations thereof may be delayed'.[17] Page actually used the word 'deferred' on this same page and perhaps this is one passage that should be considered when the novelty of Freud's concept of the deferred action of trauma (first expounded in 1896 – see Sulloway [18]) is reviewed. In my opinion the innovative element in Freud's version is that puberty changes the nature of the remembering subject in such a way as to render a childhood experience that was originally experienced neutrally, or even as pleasurable, traumatic. In other words the innovation Freud made was to claim that sexual maturation transformed the autobiographical memory of a subject. Clearly the basic view that psychical trauma may exert a deferred action and give rise to somatic symptoms was current as early as 1883 in Page's text.

Page had much more to say about the temporal aspects of nervous shock. He devoted the whole of chapter five of the book to a discussion of the many factors promoting chronicity of pain without lesion in cases of nervous shock. For the sake of clarity I shall list these, though in the text they are presented as overlapping processes:

1. Pains due to musculoskeletal sprain, felt maximally on the second or third day after the accident, 'renew the alarm of the sufferer, whose attention is thereby more closely directed to them, and their import becomes gravely aggravated in his mind.'

2. Focusing attention on the body renders sensations of normal organic functions, such as bowel contractions, conscious. These are 'unconscious' in the normal person.[19] Consciousness of these feelings leads to further introspection and so a vicious circle is perpetuated. Note here, as in the work of Holland and Carpenter, that the issues of attention (morbid introspection) amd cenesthesis are entwined. Page actually cites Maudsley and Tuke at this point, so confirming Clark's argument [20] that discussion of morbid introspection ran through many British Victorian medical authors.

3. The exaggerated painful sensations lead to the development of abnormal beliefs, such as hopelessness about the possibility of recovery, and hence disability is further prolonged.

4. The pain, by its very duration, maintains the exaggerated importance the patient attaches to it. Thus chronicity of pain in itself breeds further chronicity.

5. Idleness and unemployment lower the spirits and reduce physical fitness.

6. Unresolved compensation is often the final nail in the coffin of recovery.

Page discussed the relationship between Nervous Shock and functional nervous disorders (or neuroses). He argued that nervous shock suspends the highest intellectual functions, notably the will, and can thus precipitate neurosis. This was especially true, he believed, in those with a past history or positive family history of neurosis. Thus Page came close to equating nervous shock with conditions such as hysteria, neuralgia and hypochondria but stopped just short of stating this equivalence definitively.

This question of the relationship between 'railway spine' and hysteria was hotly debated by Page's contemporaries in Germany and France in the 1880s. Hermann Oppenheim argued for a distinction between those conditions he called 'traumatic neuroses' and hysteria, while Paul Möbius in Vienna[21] and Charcot [22] in Paris dismissed this distinction. As an aside it is interesting to note that Möbius formed the same opinion as Page regarding the 'pseudoparalysis' seen in railway cases. He coined the term *akinesia algera* for an inability to move because all or part of the body is felt to be painful.[23]

In the final chapter Page turned to the distinction between nervous shock and malingering. He was not keen on the electrical methods that had been devised in an attempt to objectify this distinction and emphasized that there were grades of dishonesty and exaggeration to be found in clinical practice. At the most obvious end of the scale would be a soldier or prisoner adding blood to his stools. In the intermediate range might be a man tempted by the possibility of financial gain to claim that an old hydrocoele had been recently caused by a railway accident or exaggerating subjective symptoms, such as pain, until compensation was settled. In the Appendix only a very few of the 234 cases Page listed were portrayed as free from the taint of malingering. Little wonder he was in such demand as an expert witness in defence of the railway companies. He was employed for over nine years as surgeon to the London and North Western Railway Company. Page was sensitive to the accusation of bias and fell back on professional independence as his defence.[24] The 'Remarks' column of the Appendix of cases reveals how wide a range of prejudices Page judged to lie within the bounds of professionalism:

Case 5: 'A nervous hysterical woman, separated from her husband. Shortly afterwards left the neighbourhood. Made an exorbitant claim.'

Case 15: 'A case of considerable exaggeration fostered by leading questions. Exorbitant claim.'

Case 21: 'A case of gross exaggeration. A total abstainer and local preacher.'

Case 30: 'A foreigner.'

Case 101: 'At the menopause.'

One final area of interest in Page's book is the brief discussion of the role of ophthalmoscopy in railway cases. Although the ophthalmoscope had been invented by Helmholtz in 1850 it was not widely used in clinical practice, at least in Britain, until the 1871 publication by Clifford Allbutt on the subject.[25] Allbutt claimed, amongst other things, that ophthalmoscopic changes were to be found accompanying injuries to the spinal cord, especially when the upper cord was involved. These changes, specifically hyperaemia and anaemia of the optic disc, were cited by Erichsen's followers in support of the notion of an organic pathophysiology of spinal concussion. Gowers and Page were less than convinced and certainly did not feel that any subtle changes in the blood supply to the retina could account for the kind of disturbances of vision that railway cases complained of, such as difficulty focusing to read.[26] Interestingly, patients seem to have got wind of the idea that their eyes were likely to be scrutinized by way of objectively assessing the veracity of their subjective complaints and Page mentions the use of atropine eye drops as a common form of malingering at this time.[27] Thus we see that the problem of pain without lesion not only attracted the most up to date theorizations – such as 'reflex inhibition' – but was also subjected to the very latest techniques of bedside examination. This is a further example of how such pain lay at the margin of clinical method and called it into question throughout the century.

Trimble [28] has described the clash between Erichsen and Page in detail but failed to offer any explanation for their divergent opinions. Perhaps the main reason that the conflict has been too readily 'solved' on the grounds that 'doctors differ' is the dating of their respective monographs. At first glance they appear contemporaneous, Erichsen 1882 versus Page 1883. However, Erichsen had been in retirement for seven years by the time the enlarged edition of his 1866 lectures was published. Page, in contrast, was 38 years old in 1883 and his book was based on his clinical work of the late 1870s. The importance of this chronology is that it reminds us that 15 years elapsed between the proposal of organic spinal concussion and Page's emphasis on psychical causes and effects. Fifteen years in which a good deal had been written about functional nervous disorders in the medical (as opposed to surgical) literature. The references in Page's work to texts from the 1870s by Allbutt, Ferrier, Gowers, Hammond, Handfield-Jones and Wilks point to a literature that had been unavailable to Erichsen in the 1860s. Moreover, Page was educated at the London Hospital in the late 1860s where one of his teachers was Hughlings Jackson. He maintained a significant interest in medicine even after specializing as a surgeon. So much so that on publication of his 1883 book he was appointed President of the Neurological Society. Thus the explanation for the difference between Erichsen and Page on 'railway spine' hinges on the latter's immersion in the new specialty of neurology. That this specialty was not yet fully established in the early 1880s is illustrated by Page, a surgeon, winning its presidency.

## 2. Pain Without Lesion in Charcot's Friday Lectures

The historiography on Charcot is now extensive and of very high quality. Most notable are Micale [29, 30,] Harris [31, 32,] Harrington [33, 34] and Noel Evans.[35] I shall refer repeatedly to these secondary sources in the course of an examination of just nine of the English translations of Charcot's 'Friday Lectures' that seem most relevant to the topic of pain without lesion. The choice of this limited primary material can be defended on grounds other than relevance. The Friday Lectures were the best prepared of Charcot's presentations and most of those I have selected were either attended, or translated into German, by Freud.

Lectures X & XI from *Lectures on the diseases of the nervous system* (published in English in 1877)[36] were delivered in the mid-1870s. This material just predates Charcot's interest in hypnosis as well as Page and Oppenheims' writings on nervous shock and traumatic neurosis. The authorities Charcot cited as he considered the phenomena of hysterical hemi-anaesthesia and ovarian hyperaesthesia were Briquet, Brodie and Skey. He regarded the chronic symptoms that persisted between hysterical fits, namely fixed pains, contractures, paralyses and hemi-anaesthesiae, as of great diagnostic value. He clearly equated the local hysteria of the British surgeons with Briquet's finding of the prevalence of left-sided pains. Charcot had a special interest in left-sided lower abdominal pain. While Briquet had called this coelialgia and regarded it as a muscle pain, Charcot dubbed it *ovarie* and attributed it to a functional lesion of the ovary:

> This would be the place to investigate what is the anatomical condition of the ovary in cases where it becomes the seat of the iliac pain of hysterical subjects...Pathological anatomy has not hitherto supplied us with any positive data in relation to this question; at present, therefore, you may designate the state of the ovary either by the term hyperkinesis, or ovarialgia, or ovaria.[37]

Such pain was described as acute, poorly localized and the ovarian region tender to palpation. Compression of the ovary reduced or stopped the hysterical fit but had no influence on the permanent symptoms of local hysteria. Five cases were then described, three of whom had exclusively left-sided symptoms.

Here we see Brodie's distinction between local and general hysteria adopted, though Charcot's description of hysterical fits, *grande hystérie,* was a more highly elaborated clinical entity than general hysteria. From Briquet came attention to the prominence of sensory symptoms in hysteria, especially pain. Micale [38] has bemoaned the overemphasis on fits in the historiography of hysteria, stating that 'the classic sensorimotor symptoms occupied pride of place in the Charcotian model of hysteria'. Shorter [39] concurs that Charcot 'upgraded [hysterical] symptoms on the sensory side' but explains this in terms of his interest in hypnotism. As I have pointed out, the study of hypnotism was a feature of Charcot's later work and in my opinion the sensory bias in his 1870s Lectures drew on Brodie and Briquet.

The conviction that hysteria had regularities just like any other neurotic disorder and was therefore amenable to precise clinical description was another part of Briquet's influence. Harris [40] has described how Charcot spoke of himself as a *visuelle,* a seer, and his contemporaries confirmed that he often scrutinized patients in complete silence. Foucault's construct of the 'medical gaze' finds its most impressive empirical support in Charcot's style, in this privileging of the visual, of inspection over anamnesis[41]. That Charcot confined himself to detailing the somatic symptoms and signs of hysteria, while downplaying, or setting aside, the psychological symptoms and mental state of the patient is understandable given his roots in pathological anatomy. Micale [42] has portrayed this somatic bias as part of an interdisciplinary 'turf war' concerning which specialty should manage hysterics. The argument is that Charcot was seeking to shift the care of hysterics from alienists, general physicians, gynaecologists and surgeons to neurologists.

So much for the early material. The second collection of Lectures I will examine were delivered between 1882 and 1885. In the years between 1875 and 1885 Charcot's ideas about hysteria evolved a good deal, largely due to his intensive study of hypnosis, though other factors, such as the rising number of compensation claims from railway and occupational accidents, played a part. Harris [43] and Harrington [44] have explored Charcot's engagement with hypnosis in detail. To summarize, a metallotherapist called Burq wrote to Bernard at the *Société de Biologie* to request that his therapeutics be formally tested. In 1876 and 1877 his work was intensively investigated on Charcot's wards at the Salpêtrière. It was found that various physical agents could move symptoms from one side of the body to the other. Metals, magnets, static electricity and electric current all seemed to do this. The phenomenon was dubbed *transfert* (transfer or transference) and the agents that mediated it *aesthesiogens.* At first only hemi-anaesthesia could be so transferred about the body, but by the mid-1880s notables such as Babinski and Féré were transferring pains and other hysterical symptoms from one side of the body to another or even from one patient to another. These pupils of Charcot felt they were actually transferring dynamic lesions from one cerebral hemisphere to the other, or from one person to the next, by means of the *aesthesiogens*. Even more extreme variations on this theme were explored by Luys at the Charité and at the Society for Psychical Research in England (founded 1882). Charcot developed strong views about hypnotism as a result of this evaluation of neo-mesmerism. Harris[45] has characterized his position as 'epiphenomenalist', that is, he regarded all the hypnotic phenomena as markers of physiological states. Only hysterics could be hypnotized and hypnotic phenomena were pathological, like the nervous system underlying them. This position was opposed from 1882 onwards by Hippolyte Bernheim in what came to be known as the Paris–Nancy debates. Bernheim had been impressed by the therapeutic value of hypnotism in the treatment of chronic pains such as neuralgias, sciatica, rheumatism and dysmenorrhoea.[46] He believed that normal persons could be hypnotized and that Charcot's linking of the phenomenon to hysteria was an irrelevance. More importantly he explained the therapeutic effects of hypnotism in terms of the action of ideas upon the body, a position Harris identifies as 'ideodynamist'. By 1884 Bernheim had come to the view that suggestion, rather than the hypnotic trance per se, was the active ingredient in these cures. This opinion won the day and was at the centre of the attacks on Charcot's *oeuvre* by many of his former pupils after his death in 1893. Babinski was one of the most prominent of these 'turncoats'.[47] He insisted that most of Charcot's findings concerning hysteria were the result of suggestion and sought to rename the condition as *pithiatism*. The importance of this story is that it allows an informed reading of Charcot's later Lectures.

Lecture I of *Clinical Lectures on Diseases of the Nervous System, Vol III* (published in English in 1889)[48] extolled the virtues of pathological anatomy:

> Pathological anatomy... furnishes to nosography more fixed, more material characters than appertain to the symptoms alone; and thus one does not fail to grasp the nature of the connections which unite the lesions to the outward signs.[49]

He then emphasized that in disorders of the nervous system the relation between structural lesion and functional disturbance can be very complex. For example, according to what he called 'the new spinal pathology' of Brown-Séquard, lesions of each region of the spinal cord gave rise to separate dysfunctions. Here he concurred with Romberg and Russell Reynolds' comments about the complex relationship between structural lesion and nervous symptom. But, in tacit opposition to Romberg, he quoted Bernard:

> Pathology should not be subordinated to physiology. Quite the reverse. Set up first the medical problem which arises from the observation of a malady, and afterwards seek for a physiological explanation. To act otherwise would be to risk overlooking the patient, and distorting the malady.[50]

Thus, for Charcot, empiricism and pathological anatomy were superior to Romberg's forced classification of the neuroses based on physiological principles. The true extent of Charcot's confidence in signs and symptoms as correlates of pathology was next revealed:

> But you are aware, gentlemen, that there still exists... a great number of morbid states, evidently having their seat in the nervous system, which leave in the dead body no material trace that can be discovered [eg. hysteria, epilepsy]... These symptomatic combinations deprived of anatomical substratum, do not present themselves to the mind of the physician with that appearance of solidity, of objectivity, which belong to affections connected with an appreciable organic lesion.[51]

He argued that such lesionless disorders have regular clinical features and that their mimickry of structural neurological diseases should be welcomed rather than feared since such 'neuromimesis' 'localises the dynamic lesion from the data furnished by an examination of the corresponding organic one.'[52] Charcot sought to localize the dynamic lesions of hysteria by sticking to exactly the same approach he had used to such good effect earlier in his career. *Lectures XX–XXII* 'On two cases of hysterical brachial monoplegia in the male' exemplify the application of this method.

In comparing the spatial distribution of altered cutaneous sensibility in the arms of Porcz and Deb, Charcot noted that in the former patient the deficit was of the whole 'arm' while in the latter it was confined exactly to the distribution of certain nerves of the brachial plexus. The first conclusion was that Porcz had an hysterical disorder while Deb was 'a typical example of a deep, old and irreparable injury of the brachial plexus'. The second conclusion was the assertion that Porcz must have a dynamic lesion of the grey matter of the cerebral hemisphere of the side opposite to the arm.[53][54]

It is the next move that Charcot made that can only be understood with reference to his studies on hypnosis. He cited Russell Reynolds on symptoms dependent upon ideas and then reproduced the pattern of Porcz's paralysis in a female hysteric by means of hypnosis. He closed the presentation with some comments on the similarities between psychic trauma and hypnotic suggestion. He argued that the emotional arousal in, say, an industrial accident put the patient into a state akin to an hypnotic trance. Then the precise point on the body that was traumatized, however slightly, was equivalent to a verbal suggestion of symptom spatialization. Under hypnosis a sharp blow to the shoulder resulted in the same symptom pattern as the hypnotist saying the word 'shoulder'.[55]

Fascinating though such a passage is, especially from the perspective of the 'prehistory of psychoanalysis', Micale [56] and Shorter [57] have emphasized that Charcot's comments on ideogenesis were a late and rather minor part of his life's work. It might be more historically correct to ask how his views on psychic trauma differed from his contemporaries Page and Oppenheim? While Page tended to use psychic trauma and nervous shock as an argument against compensation for patients, and almost universally raised the spectre of malingering in such cases, Charcot was sympathetic to the male hysterics he encountered who had developed symptoms after accidents. He also drew a sharp distinction between the phenomena of malingering and hysteria, going so far as to devise instruments to support such a contrast. For instance, in *Lecture I* he compared pressure drum tracings from hysterical and voluntary immobility of the outstretched arm.[58] Charcot also argued against Oppenheim's distinction between hysteria and 'traumatic neuroses'. For Charcot these were identical conditions, though he admitted that in traumatized men a permanent melancholia was usually seen, in contrast to female hysterics.[59]

The first two cases of male hysteria in *Lecture XVIII* further illustrate Charcot's ideas on the aetiology and symptomatology of hysteria. Rig-. was a 46-year-old ex-cooper. 'The hereditary neurosis' was 'strongly marked in his family' while the symptoms were provoked by a life-threatening accident. The 'shock' in such a case could occur with or without physical injury. In this case hemi-anaesthesia, fits, anxiety and sadness followed. Gil-., a 32-year-old metal gilder had been knifed in the head and left for dead in the street 5 years before. He now suffered left-sided hemi-anaesthesia, fits, melancholia and 'an intense cephalalgia of a peculiar character' that was made worse by reading or writing. In this case Charcot felt obliged to make a dual diagnosis of neurasthenia and hystero-epilepsy, the former being used to account for the prominent pain and melancholia. This raises the question of whether much of this exposition of Charcot's ideas on hysteria is pertinent to the topic of pain without lesion. I hope my reading of *Lectures XXIII & XXIV* 'On a case of hysterical hip disease in a man' will confirm the necessity of this lengthy overview.

Ch-. was a 45-year-old father of seven and sawyer. He exemplified the point that strong men could fall victim to hysteria, it being an ordinary disease like any other. He had been thrown into the air in an accident 3 years before and had suffered hip pain ever since, walking with crutches. Before presenting the clinical signs Charcot offered a two page summary of Brodie's views.[60] He then reported that the man displayed 'Brodie's sign' (i.e. hyperaesthetic skin over the hip joint) as well as left-sided hemi-anaesthesia to pinprick and temperature and diminution of the special senses on the left. Charcot examined the joint under chloroform anaesthesia to show there was no crepitus or limitation of movement. Next he presented two hysterical women limping with painful hips in an identical fashion to the patient. These states had been artificially created by hypnotic suggestion earlier, one by touch, the other by verbal suggestion. The conclusion was that the man's pain was an hysterical symptom and so potentially curable. Charcot closed the case presentation by informing the audience, after the patient had left the room, that the wait for compensation from the employer was perpetuating all the patient's symptoms. There was, however, no hint of malingering: the pattern of symptoms could only be the result of a dynamic lesion. This case of pain without lesion exemplifies Charcot's British influences as well as his immersion in the fields of pathological anatomy and hypnosis.

We have seen that Charcot explained lesionless pain in at least three different contexts. First were the fixed pains of permanent hysteria, such as *ovarie*. Then the invocation of neurasthenia as an explanation for pain in association with depression in men. Thirdly, hysterical pain proper as in the case of Ch-. What is most difficult to reconstruct are the grounds on which any given pain was assigned to one of these categories.

To conclude this section, it is of great interest to compare the evolution of Charcot's views on functional symptoms with that of Russell Reynolds. In 1855 Reynolds sought to explain all pains without structural lesions in terms of a functional lesion, the effects of which were mediated by the complex anatomy and physiology of the nervous system. Thus the body at play was that of neuroanatomy and neurophysiology and the interpretation of the symptom depended on the physician's knowledge of these domains. By 1869 he had come to the conclusion that another body was at stake in the tempero-spatial pattern of some pains without structural lesion: the body as imagined by the patient. Here the ideas and lay anatomical assumptions of the patient shaped the symptom. The decoding of such symptoms depended on the doctor's knowledge of the patient's ideas.[61]

Charcot traversed similar terrain in the early 1880s, allowing a version of ideogenesis a place alongside the rapidly growing understanding of localization of function in the central nervous system. Thus from the 1870s onwards the term 'functional' came to have both physiological and psychological referents in elite French and British neurological texts. But this should not be overstated. There was resistance to ideogenesis as a pathoplastic force, notably in the very influential *Manual* by Gowers[62] (see below). And Charcot never really embraced ideodynamism proper or the methodological challenges it posed. A tentative distinction should be drawn between Russell Reynolds and Charcot in their conceptions of ideogenesis. The former author seems to have offered no explanation of how ideas can provoke, sustain and shape symptoms such as pain or paralysis. Charcot, in contrast, believed that a dynamic lesion was present in the cortical domain corresponding to the region of the body implicated by the patient's ideas. To put this another way, 'having the idea that his hip hurt' was, for Charcot, just a way of saying 'having a dynamic lesion in that area of the cortex in which pain sensation from the hip is localized'. The patient's ideas were mere epiphenomena of the neurophysiology. For example, in the case of an hypnotically-induced pain being transferred from one individual to another, he sought to explain how the dynamic lesion could be so mobile rather than accepting that the transfer of ideas was primary.

We turn finally to the methodological implications of ideodynamism. If the interpretation of ideogenic symptoms depends on a detailed acquaintance with the patient's ideas about the shape and workings of his own body, then the onus is on the physician to explore the patient's views in detail. In a nutshell, the patient's subjectivity becomes the focus of inquiry and he can no longer be a silent object under the scrutiny of a largely visual medical gaze. The verbal, that is detailed history taking and idiographic investigation, now attains priority. Charcot did not respond to these methodological challenges since he never accepted ideodynamism proper. It was left to his pupils, notably Janet and, less directly, Freud to exploit this domain.

### 3. Neurasthenia in the 1880s

Now we should pause to consider the appearance of neurasthenia in the European medical literature. We have already seen that Charcot was drawing upon this diagnosis in the early 1880s, as an explanation for prominent pain and melancholic symptoms in some male patients. Oppenheim, in Vienna, was also interested in this syndrome. He particularly emphasized the nature of the low mood in neurasthenics and contrasted this with melancholia proper.[63] But it is the reception and fate of neurasthenia in Britain in the 1880s that I will explore in more detail.

Neurasthenia has attracted some historical interest, and the work of Sicherman,[64] Gosling [65] and Wessely [66] is the basis for the brief discussion presented here. George Beard coined the term in 1869 in the United States as a synonym for nervous exhaustion. The original symptom complex included fatigue, lesionless pains, hopelessness, morbid fears and low mood. In the 1870s a series of editions of *Wear and Tear* and *Fat and Blood* by Weir Mitchell promoted the rest cure and further popularized the diagnosis. With the publication of the second, and definitive, edition of Beard's *A Practical Treatise on nervous exhaustion (neurasthenia)* in 1880[67] the diagnosis crossed the Atlantic and was adopted in Europe. The gynaecologist Playfair and the physician Clifford Allbutt were among the first to write at length on the subject in England.

Playfair's *The Systematic Treatment of Nerve Prostration and Hysteria* of 1883[68] was described by the author as simply an attempt to introduce neurasthenia and the rest cure to England. However, the author was a gynaecologist while Beard and Weir Mitchell were American neurologists. Thus the opening shots of a professional demarcation dispute were fired in this otherwise innocuous monograph. Playfair described neurasthenics thus: 'Bedridden...sleepless, victims to chloral and morphia, worn and wasted, and burdens to themselves and their families'.[69] More specifically he listed the multiple somatic and moral symptoms: pain, backache, disordered menstruation, anaemia, loss of appetite, dyspepsia, emotionality, morbid selfishness, craving for sympathy. And the optimum treatment: removal from the home, that was, from 'the morbid atmosphere of invalid habits' and the 'injudicious sympathy' of family and friends, followed by feeding up with milk, six to eight weeks bedrest, passive muscular exercises (using massage and electricity) and gradual withdrawal of all drugs, especially opiates.

In the case histories of therapeutic successes, which make up the bulk of the book, Playfair emphasized the complex inter-relation between local disease of the female genitalia and the generalized 'neurotic element'.[70] The unspoken corollary of this was the need for gynaecological expertise in managing such cases. One example will suffice to illustrate this and to confirm the centrality of lesionless pain in the diagnosis of neurasthenia.

Case 4.[71] A 47-year-old single woman who had been an invalid for 10 years. She suffered painful menstrual periods and 'constant pain in the left side and back, extending down the left thigh and leg, with loss of muscular power in that side.' She was having hypodermic injections of morphine up to ten times each day. In her own words:

> I can hardly tell you what a deep sufferer and how prostrate I have been. For years I have led a completely sedentary life, always lying; it is the position I am easiest in. My back aches sorely. I am peculiarly sensitive to pain. I spend very restless nights. The pain is often then very bad.

The treatment was initially thwarted by severe morphine withdrawal symptoms but, after a change of nurse, a cure ensued. On recovery, Playfair tells us, the woman looked 20 years younger and travelled to Niagara Falls and the Cape.

Clifford Allbutt's Gulstonian Lectures to the Royal College of Physicians the following year were, in part, an angry response to Playfair's claims of expertise in the realm of neurosis. They were published in 1884 under the title *On Visceral Neuroses*.[72]

At the time of these lectures Allbutt had been a physician in Leeds for over 20 years and had considerable clinical experience with neurotics. His surgical collaborator in Leeds was the son of the T. P. Teale of spinal irritation fame (see Chapter Two above) and in 1880 he had called all the doctors in Leeds together to prevent the ugly spectacle of physicians opposing each other in court on the issue of railway spine. He had also pioneered the use of ophthalmoscopy in nervous disorders, developed techniques for hypodermic injection of morphine in chronic pain and warned against morphine addiction in neuralgics. In the years after these lectures he was first a Commissioner in Lunacy in London (1889–92), then Regius Professor of Physic at Cambridge University (see Rolleston[73] for further biographical details).

Allbutt began by summarizing four levels of pathology that could underly the symptom of dyspepsia: ulceration/tumour, gastritis, functional disturbance of the stomach and functional disturbance of the nerves innervating the stomach (neuralgia).[74] The pathophysiology in many cases lay somewhere between the latter two and the physician's role was 'to separate the pure neuralgias from the...pains of local origin'. Allbutt then turns to his main themes – the fate of the female neurotic pain patient in the hands of the gynaecologist and the distinction, crucial for him, between neuralgic/neurasthenic neurotics and hysterics. I will quote at length because these extracts are of great historical interest.

> All neuroses are commoner in women...women, speaking generally, feel pain more than men do; patient as they are, they seem to have less reserve of force and less resistance, more susceptibility and resentment, and less capacity...Men and women are variously organised in respect of resistance to pain, and their fortitude or their despair must be tested, not by their cries, but by other features of their characters. What right have we to say that a man writhing in the pangs of toothache is a great sufferer, while, in the same breath, we hint that a woman complaining of a pain in the abdomen is hysterical. The pain is equally invisible, equally unmeasured in the two cases, and the degree of credit to be given to the complaints is to be judged by other probabilities. A neuralgic woman seems thus to be peculiarly unfortunate... [she will either be labelled hysterical or referred to a gynaecologist for uterine examination] ...she is entangled in the net of the gynaecologist, who finds her uterus, like her nose, is a little on one side...so that the unhappy viscus is impaled upon a stem, or perched upon a prop, or is painted with carbolic acid every week in the year except during the long vacation when the gynaecologist is grouse-shooting, or salmon-catching...Her mind thus fastened to a mystery becomes newly apprehensive and physically introspective, and the morbid chains are riveted more strongly than ever.[75]

I will make four comments on this passage. First, and most obviously, there is the crude and hilarious professional rivalry with Playfair and his ilk. Unsurprisingly these lectures caused a good deal of controversy and it was only ten years later, as the neurasthenia diagnosis was in sharp decline, that Allbutt and Playfair could bring themselves to write a joint piece on the subject.[76] The second point of note is the discussion of pain and gender. Gosling [77] has shown that there was a one-to-one male-to-female ratio for neurasthenia in the United States. We have seen that Charcot particularly favoured the neurasthenia diagnosis in men. Here Allbutt is arguing for a female predominance of neuralgic neurotics or neurasthenics.

Thirdly, we see the issue of attention and morbid introspection raised again in the latter part of this quote. Finally, and most intriguingly, Allbutt posed the question of how to judge or measure the 'invisible' experience of pain. His answer was rather extraordinary. He advocated the use of indirect indices – 'features of their characters' – rather than the cries of pain patients themselves. At first sight this seems outrageous, to ignore the self-report of suffering. But Allbutt was simply pointing out that the doctor must make a judgement about the context from which the patient speaks (including the patient's appearance, premorbid personality, compensation issues, etc.) and would be ill-advised to take the pain words at face value.

Allbutt focused next on what he saw as a 'central blunder', the 'stupid confusion between the hysteric and the neurotic subject'. The thrust of his claim was that hysteria was very rare, even among women, and that 'neuralgia, neurosis and neurasthenia' were common. He claimed to have seen 151 cases of neurosis in 1883 alone. He then contrasted the clinical characteristics of hysterics and neuralgic neurotics/neurasthenics. Allbutt used social class as his metaphor for this distinction: 'I have endeavoured to formulate a distinction between what I may call the upper class of neurotics and their degenerate relations the hysterics'.[78] But as Sicherman[79] and Wessely [80] have argued, this metaphor was rather literally true. Neurasthenia was a diagnosis made of the upper social classes, it was seen as a disease of overwork, of civilization. It was less stigmatizing than the psychiatric diagnoses of hysteria or hypochondria and was much preferred by middle class patients and their physicians. Gosling [81] agrees that four times as many professional as working class patients were diagnosed neurasthenic (in the U.S.) but emphasizes that the diagnosis was by no means reserved for the well off. The social class gradient may be a reporting bias based on the clinical experience of a medical elite of private neurologists.

Allbutt's characterization of the hysteric and the neuralgic may actually owe as much to the metaphor of photography as to social class considerations. He referred to Mr Galton by name[82] and his descriptions of these patients very much resembles what would nowadays be included in the 'appearance and behaviour' section of a mental state examination. It was these visible, 'objective' features that Allbutt advocated be used in judging the veracity and severity of pain, as an alternative to the often misleading 'subjective' complaints of the sufferer.

The hysteric was described as:

a person of feeble purpose, limited reason, of foolish impulse, of wanton humours, of depraved appetites, of indefinite and inconsistent complaints... often fat and lazy, always selfish... capricious, listless, wilful, attractive perhaps... Such a patient is...a degenerate member of the neurotic family.[83]

While the neuralgics were 'almost the best people in this wicked world!'. Allbutt described a man with brisk step, observant eye, slightly built with hollow cheeks and temples and a sallow complexion. He has straight, fine, sparse hair and sharp features. Thin lips, dry skin (perhaps eczematous) and a narrow tongue. His fingers and wrists are bony. He is active, lively, keen, a brilliant conversationalist. He makes a reluctant patient but gives a long and accurate history of his condition and past treatments.

The case histories of Allbutt's neuralgic neurotics reveal more about his ideas on aetiology and his fascination with these patients. The first case he presented as 'typical' was of a young woman with a family history of neurosis, eccentricity and high intelligence who was 'in some degree under the stress of what Anstie called the unconscious sexual impulse'. She had been on her back for months with pelvic and abdominal pains and dysmenorrhoea. She also complained of loss of appetite and weight. On physical examination the vagina, uterus and rectum were all tender. Allbutt diagnosed 'neurosis, neuralgic type'.[84] He insisted she stand, walk and ride horses and prescribed various drugs. Within six months of this combined moral and drug therapy she was 'mixing in society' and 'riding gently to hounds'. In this case we see heredity and unconscious sexual impulses invoked as causal factors of pain without lesion. Another case report reveals the nature and extent of Allbutt's interest.

Miss -, aged 27 was seen by Allbutt in 1880. She had a neurotic family history and had suffered headaches for 9 years, provoked by mental work.

> This patient was a lady of attractions both personal and mental, and her case presented many interesting features. Her vivid perceptions, alertness... and utter unselfishness marked her as a type of the more highly endowed neurotic, and I took much interest in her case.[85]

With the benefit of hindsight we might say that Allbutt was overinvolved in this case and succumbed to the patient's 'attractions'. He certainly could not countenance the diagnosis of hysteria, that is, degeneracy for this charming patient. It is of interest that 1880 was the year in which Breuer began his intensive treatment of Anna O., another bright, young, female patient suffering neurotic pain (and other symptoms). The end of Breuer's treatment, his flight from the patient when she announced a pseudopregnancy and he realized his overinvolvement with her threatened his marriage, has become part of psychoanalytic folklore (see Hirschmüller [86]). It was probably a key source for the theorization of transference by Freud.

Despite Allbutt's enthusiasm for sparing some patients the indignity of a diagnosis of hysteria by deploying neurasthenia, the latter diagnosis was 'relegated...to the neurological dustbin' by Gowers in 1888.[87] This is not to say the term disappeared entirely. It remained in use in various ways until around 1920. For example Freud, in 1895, limited the syndrome to headaches, spinal irritation, dyspepsia and constipation.[88] Neurasthenia and the new diagnosis of anxiety neurosis were 'actual neuroses', as opposed to the 'psychoneuroses': hysteria and obsessional neurosis. The actual neuroses were caused by the patient's current sexual practices, neurasthenia being specifically attributed to masturbation, while the psychoneuroses were, he believed, rooted in sexual traumas of childhood. In French psychiatry 'hystero-neurasthenia' was still current in 1911 (see Chapter Eight below) despite Janet's concept of 'psychaesthenia' which had been 'carved out of neurasthenia'.[89] The lesson that Bynum [90] draws is that neurasthenia was one of the last lesionless nervous disorders that concerned neurologists. After 1888 the care of the nervous patient was increasingly left to psychiatrists and psychoanalysts, and this will be reflected in the professional orientation of the doctors who will figure in the remainder of this book.

### 4. Gowers on Pain

Macdonald Critchley[91] has provided a vivid biography of Gowers. We read of a man who was a product of the unique postgraduate learning environment at the newly founded National Hospital for Nervous Diseases, Queen Square. He suffered recurrent unexplained abdominal pain for eight years after starting work as Registrar there in 1870. He was influenced by Russell Reynolds and remained close to Clifford Allbutt from 1870 to 1900. He is portrayed as a highly obsessional ex-botanist, with a special interest in non-flowering plants. In 1894 he suffered 'sciatica' and a nervous breakdown of some sort. Despite the fact that the weighty second volume of his *Manual* was devoted to functional nervous disorders, Critchley states that Gowers's preference was very much for those neurological conditions where symptoms allowed precise localization of lesion.[92]

The organization of *A Manual of Diseases of the Nervous System* [93] reflected Gowers's classification of the disorders into organic, structural and functional diseases. Coarse organic diseases were visible to the naked eye, structural lesions sometimes needed a microscope. Functional diseases were dysfunctions which, he hoped, would mostly turn out to be disorders of nutrition. Be that as it may, discussion of the functional diseases was deferred to the second volume: 'The bulk of such [functional] diseases are best considered after the organic diseases have been described, since many of them are of wide distribution or uncertain seat'.[94]

In an introductory passage to Volume I on the testing of sensation, Gowers insisted on the value of testing sensibility to touch, temperature and pain separately and routinely. Distinctions between anaesthesia (loss of touch) and analgesia (loss of pain sensation) and, more importantly, hyperaesthesia and hyperalgesia were made. Romberg had certainly not made the latter distinction 40 years earlier. Gowers was more confident about this separation of pain and touch because he had now reached a firm conclusion about sensory conduction in the spinal cord. Drawing on the work of both Brown-Séquard and Schiff he stated: 'From all the evidence, direct and indirect, it seems to be almost certain that the antero-lateral ascending tract constitutes the path for sensibility to pain' and he added that tactile sensibility was conveyed in the posterior columns.[95] This is the part of Gowers's writings that has been commented upon to date by historians of pain. Keele depicts the quotation above as the culmination of the 'quest for structural equivalents for each sense'[96] while Rey praises Gowers 'for a more precise localization of these routes than that proposed by Brown-Séquard, and closer to our present-day knowledge'.[97] Meanwhile Morris complains that 'nineteenth-century researchers created the scientific basis for believing that pain was owing simply to the stimulation of specific nerve pathways', so emptying pain of all meaning and reducing it to 'no more than an electrical impulse speeding along the nerves'.[98] While Rey can be criticized on historiographic grounds for assigning praise, a more crucial objection may be levelled at Morris. He, and Merskey & Spear,[99] assume that the work of Gowers and his forerunners meant that pain was thereafter either judged to be organic or else dismissed as imaginary. Here these historians entirely gloss over his writings on functional nervous disorders. It is to the second volume of the *Manual* that we must now turn to correct this.

Lesionless pain was discussed in passages on neuralgia, headache, hysteria and hypochondriasis. Gowers advocated that the term 'neuralgia' be reserved only for cases without primary organic lesions of the nerve trunk. Thus many of the cases that Romberg and Anstie had included were now excluded from the category and had been discussed in Volume I as 'neuritis'. The discussion of the causes of neuralgia immediately makes clear that Morris's depiction of Gowers' views on pain is inaccurate:

> A lady was intensely distressed after parting with her husband, who was going to America. She felt on the point of bursting into tears, and as if the tears would give her relief. Her sister said, 'Do not cry; you shall not cry'. By an effort she succeeded in restraining her tears, but was immediately conscious of a sense of intense pressure above the eyebrows, and a few days later severe supra-orbital neuralgia came on upon the left side, and lasted for several weeks.[100]

Now far from dismissing such pain of emotional origin as imaginary, Gowers suggests that the pain is due to dysfunction of the central nervous system, perhaps the dorsal root ganglia. His evidence for this localization of invisible dysfunction was the phenomena of irradiation and reflexion. The former named the spread of pain beyond the distribution of an individual sensory nerve while the latter described pain felt in quite another region than an irritated nerve.

He divided and redivided the neuralgias by their 'situation' (trigeminal, brachial, visceral etc) and their 'character' (herpetic, diabetic, anaemic, hysterical, syphilitic etc). This complex taxonomy does not detract from the fact that he actually narrowed the referent of the term compared to Anstie. Alam & Merskey [101] had difficulty explaining their finding that neuralgia's meaning contracted substantially in the 1880s. I suspect Gowers's clear distinction between neuritis and neuralgia was very influential in this respect.

Headache could be diagnosed as migrainous, neuralgic, neurasthenic or hysterical. In addition to definite pains of the head Gowers discussed

> 'Head pressure and other cephalic sensations'. Various bizarre sensations, not as simple as pain which the patient, in default of adequate terms, describes by some simile beyond the range of ordinary experience, such as 'a feeling as if the brains were being stirred up with a stick'... or 'as if the head were being alternately opened and shut'... The chief agency in the production of these sensations is certainly the mental state of the patient.[102]

In this passage Gowers is distinguishing lesionless pains from lesionless sensations of greater complexity described by the patient in metaphorical language. He was quick to ascribe the former to dysfunction of specific parts of the central nervous system while these latter phenomena were, he argued, part of mental illness. It seems as if the patient's use of subjective language led the neurologist to diagnose subjective sensation. Gowers called these idiosyncratic sensations 'receptive dysaesthesiae'. In the later French psychiatric literature these phenomena were discussed under the rubric of 'cenestopathy', and Blondel in particular had a lot to say about the relationship between subjectivity and language (see Chapter Eight).

'Hysteria is probably the most perfect type of a functional malady' wrote Gowers, and a 43-page discussion followed. He cited Russell Reynolds, Briquet and Charcot on the subject and drew attention to heredity and emotional disturbance as predisposing and precipitating causes respectively. Gowers added a list of mental state abnormalities to the continuous or permanent somatic symptoms of hysteria that Brodie, Briquet and Charcot had described. Impulsivity, irritability, self-centredness and the use of exagerrated description of symptoms were all characteristic. Complaints of pain were hard to judge in such patients:

> The nervous system is dominated by ideas, as well as by emotions; the definite conception of a symptom may lead to its occurrence; and when idea and emotion are conjoined, and a symptom is not only conceived but either dreaded or desired, its occurrence is still more easy... if a definite pain is thought of, before long it may be felt, without the symptom being in any case intentionally induced... It is often difficult to learn how far there is an actual increase of sensation and how far the exaggeration is in the description of the feeling.[103]

He closed the section with the observation that local pains and hemi-anaesthesia were much harder to relieve than the motor symptoms in hysteria. Breuer had found the same with Anna O. but suppressed the persistence of her facial pain in his published case history of 1895.[104]

Gowers's definition of hypochondriasis placed the emphasis on the mood and beliefs of the patient rather than their perceptions. This was in contrast to early nineteenth-century authors who rather dwelt on aberrant sensation as the core of the problem. The explanation for this shift is not obvious, though the new psychiatric literature on the delusions of Melancholics (e.g. Clouston – see Chapter Seven below) may have influenced Gowers, since the differential diagnosis between primary hypochondriasis and the hypochondriacal delusions of melancholics was clearly his main concern:

Hypochondriasis is a morbid state of the nervous system in which there is mental depression due to erroneous ideas of such bodily ailments as might conceivably be present. This limitation is necessary to distinguish the condition from those forms of actual insanity in which there is a delusion of the existence of some impossible ailment – impossible in its nature or else by reason of its incompatability with life.[105]

Thus, for Gowers, worries about silent bowel cancer implied hypochondriasis while 'my brains are made of sawdust' was seen as a melancholic delusion. Here, as in the distinction between headache and metaphorical descriptions of dysaesthesias, the speech of the patient held the key to diagnosis.

### Summary

In Chapter Five we saw that Briquet listed heredity, the sexual life of the individual and psychic traumas as the three main causes of Hysteria. In Chapter Six I have shown how these factors, and especially the third of them, attracted a great deal of attention in writings on functional nervous disorders of the 1870s and 1880s. Psychic trauma was discussed at length by Page, Charcot and Gowers. The equivalence of the shock of an accident and hypnotic trance, the deferred action of psychic trauma, the equivalence of verbal and tactile suggestions to hypnotized or traumatized subjects, the relative importance of ideas and emotions in the aetiology of neuroses – all these were explored. And yet none of the authors embraced ideogenesis without interposing a dysfunctional nervous system between idea and symptom. In Chapter Seven we shall see that this was also the case in the writings of psychiatrists of the period.

We have seen how efforts were made to rescue neuralgic or neurasthenic neurotics from the category of degenerate hysterics using judgements based on social class, premorbid personality and general physical appearance. This option was closed in 1888 when Gowers dismissed neurasthenia and narrowed the meaning of the term neuralgia considerably. Henceforth patients with lesionless pains other than classical tic douloureux were of less interest to neurologists and more likely to be directed to psychiatrists. This will be reflected in the choice of primary sources in the remainder of my book.

Finally, there was clearly increasing attention to the use of language by pain patients in the 1880s. For example, Gowers began to ask whether the problem lay at the level of pain perception or pain description in cases of lesionless pain. The use of unusual metaphors by those complaining of pain in the absence of structural pathology was now taken as a sign of insanity, psychosis, while orthodox pain language in the absence of lesion pointed to neurosis. In Chapter Eight we shall see how this line of thought reached its climax in the work of a number of French alienists.

## Notes

1. Erichsen, 1882, *On concussion of the spine, nervous shock and other obscure injuries of the nervous system.*
2. *Ibid.,* 2.
3. Trimble, 1981, *Post-traumatic neurosis: from railway spine to the whiplash.*
4. Erichsen, 1882, 14, *On concussion of the spine, nervous shock and other obscure injuries of the nervous system.*
5. *Ibid.* 15.
6. *Ibid.,* 104–6.
7. *Ibid.,* 20–23.
8. Hilton, 1863, 54–7, *On the influence of mechanical and physiological rest in the treatment of accidents and surgical diseases, and the diagnostic value of pain.*
9. Skey, 1867, 83, *Hysteria.*
10. Page, 1883, *Injuries of the spine and spinal cord without apparent mechanical lesion, and nervous shock, in their surgical and medico-legal aspects.*
11. *Ibid.,* 86–8.
12. *Ibid.,* 111.
13. *Ibid.,* 128–9.
14. *Ibid.,* 158–66.
15. *Ibid.,* 145.
16. *Ibid.,* 147.
17. *Ibid.* 148.
18. Sulloway, 1992, 111, *Freud, biologist of the mind: beyond the psychoanalytic legend.*
19. Page, 1883, 175, *Injuries of the spine and spinal cord without apparent mechanical lesion, and nervous shock, in their surgical and medico-legal aspects.*
20. Clark, 1988, *Morbid introspection, unsoundness of mind, and British psychological medicine c. 1830 – c. 1900.*
21. Schiller, 1982, *A Möbius strip: fin-de-siècle neuropsychiatry and Paul Möbius.*
22. Charcot, 1889, 221–5, *Clinical lectures on diseases of the nervous*

*system, Volume III.*

23. Schiller, 1982, *A Möbius strip: fin-de-siècle neuropsychiatry and Paul Möbius.*

24. Page, 1883, preface, *Injuries of the spine and spinal cord without apparent mechanical lesion, and nervous shock, in their surgical and medico-legal aspects.*

25. Spillane, 1981, 354, *The doctrine of the nerves: chapters in the history of neurology.*

26. Page, 1883, 191–3, *Injuries of the spine and spinal cord without apparent mechanical lesion, and nervous shock, in their surgical and medico-legal aspects.*

27. *Ibid.,* 231–2.

28. Trimble, 1981, *Post-traumatic neurosis: from railway spine to the whiplash.*

29. Micale, 1990(b) *Charcot and the idea of hysteria in the male.*

30. Micale, 1994, *Charcot and les névroses traumatiques: historical and scientific reflections.*

31. Harris, 1985, *Murder under hypnosis in the case of Gabrielle Bompard: psychiatry in the courtroom in Belle Époque Paris.*

32. Harris, 1991, Introduction to Charcot's *Clinical lectures on diseases of the nervous system.*

33. Harrington, 1987, *Medicine, mind and the double brain.*

34. Harrington, 1988, *Hysteria, hypnosis and lure of the invisible: the rise of neo-mesmerism in fin-de-siècle French psychiatry.*

35. Noel Evans, 1991, *Fits and starts: a genealogy of hysteria in modern France.*

36. Charcot, 1877 *Lectures on the diseases of the nervous system.*

37. *Ibid.,* 269.

38. Micale, 1990(b) *Charcot and the idea of hysteria in the male.*

39. Shorter, 1992, 150, *From paralysis to fatigue: a history of psychosomatic illness in the modern era.*

40. Harris, 1991, Introduction. In *Clinical lectures on diseases of the nervous system.*

41. It is, however, possible to overstate the primacy of the "medical gaze" in French hospital medicine. Although Charcot relied on inspection, his later case histories, on male hysteria dating from the 1880s, include historical detail, especially concerning family history and details of any accident involving the patient. Jacyna (1995) has suggested that the empiricist bias of Paris medicine may have been at the level of professional rhetoric rather than praxis. For example, Alibert, the Paris physician best known as the father of dermatology, included lengthy personal histories alongside illustrations of skin

conditions in his books (circa 1815), and even documented these patients' views on the causes of their own diseases. This casts some doubt on Foucault's bold generalisation.

42. Micale 1990 (b) *Charcot and the idea of hysteria in the male.*
43. Harris, 1985, *Murder under hypnosis in the case of Gabrielle Bompard: psychiatry in the courtroom in Belle Époque Paris.*
44. Harrington, 1987, *Medicine, mind and the double brain.*
45. Harris, 1985, *Murder under hypnosis in the case of Gabrielle Bompard:.*
46. *Ibid.*, 208.
47. Noel Evans, 1991, *Fits and starts: a genealogy of hysteria in modern France.*
48. Charcot, 1889, Lecture I, Clinical lectures on diseases of the nervous system, Volume III.
49. *Ibid.*, 10.
50. *Ibid.*, 8.
51. *Ibid.*, 12.
52. *Ibid.*, 14.
53. *Ibid.*, Lecture XX–XXII, 278.
54. While Brodie and Skey had commented on the non-anatomical distribution of pains in hysteria, Charcot could present this phenomenon in much more detail due to the advances in neurological theory and bedside examination. For example, the cases analysed here depended on knowledge of decussation as well as a distinction between analgesia and absolute anaesthesia (Charcot 1889, p 269).
55. *Ibid.*, 304.
56. Micale, 1990 (b) *Charcot and the idea of hysteria in the male.*
57. Shorter, 1992, *From paralysis to fatigue: a history of psychosomatic illness in the modern era.*
58. Charcot, 1889, Lecture I, 16–17, *Clinical lectures on diseases of the nervous system.*
59. *Ibid.*, Lecture XXII, 224–5.
60. *Ibid.*, Lecture XXIII & XXIV, 320–1.
61. The question of which body is at stake in hysteria was raised by David-Ménard (1989). Her difficult, but stimulating book is further considered in Chapter Seven.
62. Gowers, 1886 & 1888, *A manual of diseases of the nervous system.*, Vol. I & II.
63. Wessely, 1990, *Old wine in new bottles: neurasthenia and 'M.E.'*
64. Sicherman, 1977, *The uses of a diagnosis: doctors, patients and neurasthenia.*

65. Gosling, 1987, *Before Freud: neurasthenia and the American medical community, 1870–1910.*

66. Wessely, 1990, *Old wine in new bottles: neurasthenia and 'M.E.'*

67. Beard, 1880, *A practical treatise on nervous exhaustion.*

68. Playfair, 1883, *The systematic treatment of nerve prostration and hysteria.*

69. *Ibid.*, 11.

70. *Ibid.*, 45.

71. *Ibid.*, 34–41.

72. Allbutt, 1884, *On visceral neuroses; being the Gulstonian Lectures on neuralgia of the stomach and allied disorders.*

73. Rolleston 1929, *The Right Hon. Sir Thomas Clifford Allbutt: a memoir.*

74. Allbutt, 1884, 7–8, *On visceral neuroses.*

75. *Ibid.*, 16–17.

76. Rolleston, 1929, 87, *The Right Hon. Sir Thomas Clifford Allbutt: a memoir.*

77. Gosling, 1987, *Before Freud: neurasthenia and the American medical community, 1870–1910.*

78. Allbutt, 1884, 30, *On visceral neuroses.*

79. Sicherman, 1977, *The uses of a diagnosis: doctors, patients and neurasthenia.*

80. Wessely, 1990, *Old wine in new bottles: neurasthenia and 'M.E.'*

81. Gosling, 1987, *Before Freud: neurasthenia and the American medical community, 1870–1910.*

82. Allbutt, 1884, 22, *On visceral neuroses.*

83. *Ibid.*, 21.

84. *Ibid.*, 25–7.

85. *Ibid.*, 40–41.

86. Hirschmüller, 1989, 95–132, *The life and work of Josef Breuer: physiology and psychoanalysis.*

87. Bynum, 1985, *The nervous patient in eighteenth- and nineteenth-century Britain: the psychiatric origins of British neurology.*

88. Wessely, 1990, *Old wine in new bottles: neurasthenia and 'M.E.'*

89. Berrios, 1985, *Obsessional disorders during the nineteenth century: terminological and classificatory issues.*

90. Bynum, 1985, *The nervous patient in eighteenth- and nineteenth-century Britain: the psychiatric origins of British neurology.*

91. Critchley, 1949, *Sir William Gowers 1845–1915: a biographical appreciation.*

92. *Ibid.*, 79–80,

93. Gowers, 1886 & 1888, *A manual of diseases of the nervous system.,*

Vol I & II.
94. *Ibid.*, Vol I, 2.
95. *Ibid.*, 130–35.
96. Keele, 1957, 10, *Anatomies of pain.*
97. Rey, 1993, 233, *History of pain.*
98. Morris, 1991, 4, *The culture of pain.*
99. Merskey & Spear, 1967, *Pain: psychological and psychiatric aspects.*
100. Gowers, 1888 736, *A manual of diseases of the nervous system.*, Vol II.
101. Alam & Merskey, 1994, *What's in a name? the cycle of change in the meaning of neuralgia.*
102. Gowers, 1888, *A manual of diseases of the nervous system*, Vol II.
103. *Ibid.*, 908–9
104. Hirschmüller, 1989, *The life and work of Josef Breuer: physiology and psychoanalysis.*
105. Gowers, 1888, 954–5, *A manual of diseases of the nervous system.*, Vol II.

# 7

## Psychalgia and Conversion:

## Pain Without Lesion in late nineteenth-century Psychiatric and Psychoanalytic Writings: 1872–1895

We have seen how the distinction between neurogenic and ideogenic pain, proposed by Russell Reynolds in 1869, was fleshed out by Charcot in the 1880s. Yet a diseased nervous system, a dynamic lesion, was always interposed between the idea and the pain symptom in Charcot's version of ideodynamism. Did those medical authors we can crudely characterize as psychiatrists or psychoanalysts embrace ideodynamism proper and explore lesionless pain in the context of the patient's detailed autobiography in the hope of explaining it? In this chapter I shall argue that Meynert and Breuer in Germany, and Tuke and Clouston in Britain, did nothing of the sort. Rather, they stuck to psychophysiological accounts of the aetiology of pain without structural lesion. Even Freud, who began to question the meaning of lesionless pain for the individual patient, clung to a psychophysiological version of ideodynamism as late as 1895.

### 1. Tuke

In 1853 Daniel Hack Tuke resumed work at the asylum his family had founded in York, after studying medicine at St Bartholomew's Hospital. Five years later the *Manual of Psychological Medicine* that he co-authored with Bucknill was published and soon was acknowledged to be the standard British text on the subject. In the following year, 1859, he became ill with pulmonary tuberculosis and was forced into medical retirement in Falmouth, where he remained until starting a private practice in London in 1875. The *Illustrations of the influence of the mind upon the body in health and disease designed to elucidate the action of the imagination*[1] were compiled between 1869 and 1872, in response to his fascination with the effects of a railway collision according to the preface. This text is therefore the work of an invalid who had not practised clinically for well over a decade.

The explicit aim of the book was to present a 'collection of psycho-physical phenomena' to promote and legitimate 'psycho-therapeutics'.[2] Two chapters included discussion of lesionless pain.

Chapter II, 'Influence of the intellect on sensation', opened with the words:

> The intellect may excite ordinary Sensations, may suspend them altogether (anaesthesia), or may induce excessive and morbid sensations (hyperaesthesia and dysaesthesia).[3]

He cited Hunter and Müller in speculating about the mechanism by which focusing attention on a part of the body may give rise to a pain-like feeling in that part. Braid and Gregory's reports of suggested sensation in hypnotized subjects were mentioned. But the sensation provoked by attention or suggestion was not quite an actual pain, according to Tuke. Neuralgias provided an example of how actual pains could be triggered by mental states. In neuralgias 'a stimulus acting centrally upon the sensory nerves' provoked pain. For example, a man felt a pain in his arm for two days after watching someone else being bled. Here the direct cause of the lesionless neuralgic pain was the mental state, that is, the ideas formed as a result of such a spectacle.[4]

Later in the chapter Tuke turned to the question of whether mere remembrance can provoke a sensation with the same qualities as pain perception. He concluded that in both perception and in recollection it is difficult to separate what he called 'ideational' and 'sensational' elements of the experience. Recollected pains will be fainter than perceived pains unless the nervous system is over-excited. When the nervous system is morbidly excited, and recollected pain is indistinguishable from perceived pain, the result is an hallucination of pain:

> In some conditions of the encephalic centres, such a powerful excitement of the sensory ganglia occurs, that the effect is identical in sensory force – in objectivity – with that which results from an impression produced upon the peripheral termination of the nerves, causing hallucinations or phantasmata.[5]

In Chapter VII 'Influence of the emotions upon sensation', Tuke argued that if ideas, unaccompanied by emotion, can give rise to pain without lesion, then:

> how much more profoundly will an intense emotion, as Fear or Joy?... Our starting point then is this: Emotional impulses may act upon the sensory ganglia and nucleii of the nerves of sensation, so as to produce any of those sensations which are ordinarily induced by impressions upon their periphery ; such sensations, although central,

160

being referred by the mind to the peripheral termination of the nerve.[6]

So Tuke, like Müller 40 years before, saw ideas, memories and emotions as physiological stimuli that may act centrally to excite sensations. Such sensations are then referred to the periphery by the law of eccentricity. It is important to stress that this was not what we now call ideogenesis at all, but was a psycho-physiological explanation for clinical phenomena. There was no direct link from idea to symptom in Tuke's model. A disordered nervous system was always interposed.

Now Clark has argued that psychiatrists like Tuke amassed a 'considerable body of Victorian medicopsychological "insights" into unconscious or abnormal mentation'[7] but could not use these as the basis for a psychotherapeutics. For them, examples of mind–body interaction always reflected a morbid nervous system and, as a morbid product, the content was unworthy of detailed interpretation. Any therapeutic use of suggestion would merely reinforce what was already a pathological phenomenon. Thus the insistent presence of a diseased brain at the root of mental phenomena, the somaticist bias, in these writings ruled out the possibility of taking psychopathological content seriously. The presence of certain psychopathological forms, such as hallucinated pain, was simply a marker of a diseased brain. My reading of Tuke on pain without lesion supports Clark's argument.

## 2. Clouston and Meynert

The compilatory work of an isolated invalid, Tuke's *Illustrations* were written under very different circumstances than those in which Thomas Clouston worked. Beveridge [8] has written an excellent introduction to his life and work. In the 1880s Clouston was at the pinnacle of his career. He was the superintendent of the most prestigious asylum in Scotland – the Royal Edinburgh Asylum – and was lecturing at the University as well as writing prolifically. Clouston encountered pain without lesion among asylum inpatients rather than in books written by others. The commonest clinical scenario was complaints of pain among melancholics. He had a theory to explain the association between melancholia and physical pains. His alternative name for melancholia in the *Clinical Lectures on Mental Diseases* of 1883[9] was 'psychalgia', and this gives us the clue. He regarded physical and mental pain as sharing an identical physiological basis. This idea was fully developed in an 1886 paper in the British Medical Journal: 'The relationship of bodily and mental pain'.[10]

The paper sought to explain a number of clinical phenomena by means of Meynert's theory of pain as expressed in his 1884 book *Psychiatry: a clinical treatise on diseases of the fore-brain*.[11] Meynert held that identical cortical states underlay bodily and mental pains. Consciousness of physical pain was the result of intense inhibition of reflex irradiation in the brain. Such inhibition impaired thought and activity. Reminiscence of pain caused an identical inhibition. This was mental pain. The brain has a certain capacity for pain, and this can be used up in bodily or mental expression. Clouston asserted that Meynert's theory held the field in 1886. It seems clear that Meynert had followed Griesinger in arguing for the equivalence of bodily pain and melancholia (see Chapter Four above). This persistence of Romantic monism with respect to pain was driven by the abundant clinical evidence of an intimate relationship between chronic pain and melancholia. Clouston's paper lists several clinical phenomena that, he believed, supported Meynert's monist theory. He noted that neuralgia often preceded bouts of melancholia and disappeared with the onset of the latter. This was called 'Circular Neurosis'. Chronic pain frequently provoked melancholia and odd bodily pains often accompanied melancholia. Neuralgia and melancholia tended to run together in families with neuropathic heredity and both neuralgics and melancholics tended to be thin individuals with little sexual feeling. Finally he had heard patients remark that visceral pain often heralded the onset of a further bout of melancholia in recurrent cases.

Meynert, and his followers such as Clouston, have often been depicted as dualists or, at best, epiphenomenalists with respect to mind–body philosophy. For example Clark[12] has argued that their fundamental view that mental disease was merely a manifestation of brain disease led them to dismiss the psychopathological products of the diseased organ as of little interest. Meynert is seen as the exemplar of an unhelpful somaticist bias in late-nineteenth-century psychiatry. Yet with respect to pain it is clear he was a monist. I shall now suggest that it was thanks to this monist view of pain in Meynertian physiology that Freud was able to conceive the notion of conversion of energy between mental and physical realms.

### 3. Freud, Breuer and 'Conversion'.

1895 was the year that Freud, in his own words, 'hit on the neuroses'.[13] It was an eventful year in which he saw the publication of *Studies on Hysteria*,[14] had the dream of Irma's injection and wrote the manuscript later known as the *Project for a Scientific Psychology*.[15] I shall limit my examination of Freud's writings to this one year and argue that these three famous Freudian texts all bear the marks of a decade of struggle on his part with the problem of pain without lesion. Of course, Freud returned to the topic of pain in later years, for example in *The Economic Problem of Masochism*,[16] but, as David-Ménard has shown, he largely lost interest in the somatic symptoms of hysterics in favour of their fantasies after 1895.[17]

According to Sulloway, Freud turned from pure physiology to medicine of necessity, and qualified in 1881. He decided to specialize in neuropathology and worked in Meynert's Laboratory for Cerebral Anatomy from 1883 until 1886, later describing Meynert as one of the most brilliant men he had ever met.[18] Meanwhile, a Viennese general practitioner rather older than Freud, Josef Breuer, was treating a patient named Bertha Pappenheim in an unusually intensive fashion, seeing her almost daily from 1880 to 1884. Breuer shared this unusual experience in detail with the younger physician. As Hirschmüller's excellent reconstruction makes clear, Pappenheim (later written up as 'Anna O.') suffered severe facial pain that was unrelieved by the 'talking cure' Breuer was pioneering, and this persistent pain was the major reason she was hospitalized after Breuer had relieved her multiple motor symptoms with psycho-therapy.[19] Thus Freud was simultaneously exposed to Meynert's view of the radical equivalence of psychic and physical pain and to Breuer's clinical finding that neuralgic pain was unrelieved by the talking cure.

In 1884 Freud himself was actively engaged in the treatment of pain by means of cocaine. His paper on the medicinal use of cocaine was published during that year. Freud was aware that many chronic pain patients became addicted to morphine and he found cocaine useful both as an analgesic and as a replacement for morphine in those who had become addicted to the latter. One of his colleagues, Fleischl von Markow, was in the predicament of morphine dependence superimposed on chronic pain from a neuroma. Freud recommended the cocaine he had found so helpful but Fleischl injected it, rather than using it nasally, and Freud felt this contributed to his premature death in 1891.[20, 21] So Freud was discovering for himself the pitfalls of medical management of chronic pain at the same time as hearing about the failure of psychotherapy for this symptom.

The following year he visited Charcot where he saw, and subsequently translated, some 'Friday Lectures'. As we have seen, these included cases of hysterical pain which Charcot demonstrated were ideogenic and thus potentially curable by hypnotic suggestion. One can imagine the enthusiasm with which Freud received these ideas and this was reflected in his rather overzealous presentation 'On Male Hysteria' to the Viennese Society of Physicians in 1886.[22]

In the late-1880s Freud came to favour Bernheim's theory of hypnosis over Charcot's less psychological model, translating one of Bernheim's books into German and visiting him briefly in Nancy in 1889. By now Freud was using hypnosis to elicit reminiscences from hysterics, as Breuer had done earlier in the decade, rather than making therapeutic suggestions. In 1892 he abandoned hypnosis in favour of allowing 'Elisabeth von R.', a chronic pain sufferer, to 'free associate' while he applied pressure to her forehead. One could therefore claim that the first patient treated psychoanalytically was a case of lesionless pain.

If we now turn to the *Studies on Hysteria*[23] we can examine Freud's ideas on pain without lesion in the early 1890s. I shall contrast his case history of Elisabeth von R. with Breuer's *Theoretical* chapter. By the time this book was published the views of the co-authors were rapidly parting company. This has been attributed to various factors, notably Breuer's reluctance to accept sexual traumas as the exclusive cause of hysteria and the differing personalities of the collaborators.[24,][25] I shall confine myself to drawing out their differences on the subject of pain without lesion.

Freud clearly believed that many lesionless pains were hysterical symptoms of psychic origin, caused by repressed reminiscences, that could be abolished by cathartic speech. The case of Elisabeth von R. affords an example. She was 24 and had suffered pains in her legs, with consequent astasia-abasia, for two years by the time she met Freud.

> The pain was of an indefinite character...a fairly large, ill-defined area of the anterior surface of the right thigh was indicated as the focus..from which they [the pains] most often radiated.[26]

But in addition to this non-anatomical localization of the pain, her reaction to pressure or pinching of her legs was 'one of pleasure rather than pain...it was as though she was having a voluptuous tickling sensation – her face flushed, she threw back her head and shut her eyes and her body bent backwards.'[27] However, there were some physical signs suggestive of 'muscular rheumatism' so Freud 'proceeded on the assumption that the disorder was of this mixed kind' (that is, part organic, part ideogenic). Although her autobiography was a sad one, Freud could not pinpoint a psychical trauma that precipitated the pain until Elisabeth told him a story about a young man she fancied. One evening she had accompanied this man to an exciting party but on returning home was confronted by a deterioration in the condition of her sick father, whom she had been nursing for some time. Freud concluded that she had repressed her erotic feelings in reponse to this conflict. This repressed affect then revived or intensified the old pain of the rheumatism. Freud called this 'the mechanism of conversion' from psychical conflict to somatic symptom.

However, this preliminary formulation had to be abandoned in favour of a stronger storyline later in the talking treatment with this woman. She came to realize that she had been in love with her sister's husband for many years. On the occasion of her sister's death her first fleeting thought had been that her brother-in-law was now free and she could marry him. Freud now proposed an alternative conversion: 'She succeeded in sparing herself the painful conviction that she loved her sister's husband, by inducing physical pains in herself instead.'[28] Conversion from the realm of psychic conflict to somatic symptom was a problem and a mystery for him – 'I cannot, I must confess, give any hint of how a conversion of this kind is brought about.'[29] In fact, Freud then appeared to back away from any claim about ideogenic pain:

> somatic pain was not *created* by the neurosis, but merely used, increased and maintained by it. I may add at once that I have found a similar state of things in almost all the instances of hysterical pains into which I have been able to obtain an insight.[30]

Having said this he immediately gave a series of brief clinical examples that entirely contradicted this cautious stance. In the case of Frau Cäcilie, facial pain was caused by a rebuff she had perceived 'like a slap in the face'[31] and pain in the foot arose from concern that she might fail to 'find herself on a right footing' with some strangers.[32] Thus Freud oscillated between accepting ideogenesis of de novo hysterical pains and insisting on their organic roots.

The most penetrating commentary on this long case history is by David-Ménard.[33] She claims that Freud's first theory of conversion was premised on mind–body dualism. She emphasizes that it was the Janus-faced use of the same word for both physical and mental pains that allowed the slippage that made conversion plausible:

> A single word, 'pain' (*schmerz*), has the function of rendering the two independent orders homogeneous so that the passage from one to the other may occur.[34]

Though David-Ménard points this out well, she does not mention the historical continuity between Meynert's monist view of pain and Freud's adoption of the same.

David-Ménard then goes on to critique any simplistic model of a one-to-one relation between words and somatic symptoms. She draws on the thought of Lacan to argue that the body at stake in hysterical symptoms is an imaginary, erotogenic one, conforming to lay beliefs about anatomy and erogenized by the lived history of the patient. She criticizes Freud for trying to reconcile the body of anatomy/physiology with the patient's speech rather than embracing the idea of an alternative body.

If we now turn to Breuer's *Theoretical* chapter we find a different position regarding neurotic pains. He emphasized that not all hysterical phenomena are ideogenic. Such pains as are ideogenic are hallucinations and, as such, are only vivid if the nervous apparatus concerned with pain sensation is dysfunctioning or over-excited. Thus apparently ideogenic phenomena actually have a clear organic basis. Breuer was here invoking the by-now traditional functional lesion of the nervous system. He conceded that pain in a joint after minor injury could be intensified or prolonged by concentration of attention on the part, 'But this can hardly be expressed by saying that the hyperalgesia has been caused by ideas'.[35] While Freud was accepting ideogenic pain by means of Meynertian monism, Breuer was strictly dualist and insisted that functional lesions must accompany somatic pains.

Freud's dream of Irma's injection, that was so central to *The Interpretation of Dreams*,[36] occurred in 1895 and throws further light on the nature and extent of his concerns about the problem of pain in that year. The dream began with a female patient whose pains persisted despite psychoanalytic interpretation, or 'my "solution"' as Freud put it:

> I said to her: 'If you still get pains, it's really only your fault.' She replied: 'If you only knew what pains I've got now...'...I was alarmed and looked at her...I thought to myself that after all I must be missing some organic trouble.

Freud was anxious about missing a lesion in a case of pain. He next reverted to medical examination, inspection of her face and throat, abandoning analytic technique. He made her open her mouth 'properly', an ambiguous phrase which refers both to overcoming her resistance to free association and to physical examination. He then involved medical colleagues in the dream but was rather critical of them. The injection later in the dream reminded him of the catastrophe that had arisen through drug treatment of chronic pain in the case of Fleischl von Markow. Freud seems to have been reminding himself that the side effects of medical treatment can be much more damaging than the incomplete cure of pain by psychoanalysis.

Finally, as Lacan points out in Seminar II[37], the 'navel' of the dream concerned anxiety, as represented by the fearful sight of the turbinate bones covered in visible lesions that he saw in Irma's throat. This anxiety concerned the financial and physical wellbeing of Freud's wife and children as he abandoned the relative security of a medical career in favour of analytic practice. But at a deeper level, Lacan argues, a premonition of his own mode of death was at play.

The importance of the dream for our purposes is that it supports the view that the topic of chronic pain, its causes, and its treatment by drugs or psychotherapy, was of vital concern to Freud in 1895 as he abandoned the medical gaze in favour of the analytic ear.

The *Project for a Scientific Psychology*[38] provides the third source for Freud on pain in 1895. Knight[39] has depicted this text as a direct response to Breuer's theoretical contribution to the *Studies on Hysteria*, which Freud had found unsatisfactory. It is a hugely complex piece of work and lengthy summaries and commentaries are available.[40, 41] The clinical phenomenon of hysterical conversion was the central problem it explored.

Freud proposed that physical pain, *schmerz*, was the result of large external energies, Q, impacting on perceptual neurones, ø neurones. His problem was to explain how, in hysteria, mere reminiscence of pain could be as vivid as the pain of current injury. He invoked two more classes of neurones to achieve this. Mnemic neurones, $\psi$, and a type of neurone concerned with qualitative aspects of experience, $\omega$, that lent 'indications of reality'.

In the healthy individual, although past pains had seared a path through certain key $\psi$ neurones and thus a memory of the pain at a neuronal level existed, the evocation of this memory was unaccompanied by any effects on ø neurones and hence no vivid pain percept resulted. The reason that reminiscence had no effect on ø neurones was that the healthy individual had a network of side routes in the mnemic $\psi$ neurones that dissipated the energy of the key $\psi$ neurones, so there was no increase in the energy in ø neurones on remembering. This inhibitory network of side routes was called the healthy ego. In the hysteric this inhibitory network in the mnemic system did not exist. Instead, defence was sought by shifting energy from the traumatic memory to a symbolically associated one. Thus charged key neurones existed, but the cue for reminiscence had changed. When the key neurones were triggered, now by a seemingly irrelevant environmental cue, there was a rise in energy in both ø and ω systems, indications of reality were present and a vivid pain hallucination was felt. However, in this model Freud equivocated about whether the pain under consideration was psychic or physical. He introduced a strange term *unlust*, or unpleasure, to complement *schmerz*. A rise in energy in ω neurones resulted in *unlust*, a rise in energy in ø neurones led to *schmerz*.

As is probably apparent, even this small fragment of the *Project* that I have presented is very complicated and, at times, unsatisfactory. Freud never sought to publish this work. Its value for us is the further evidence it provides of the great stimulus and difficulty pain without lesion posed to theorization at this time.

To conclude, a range of textual material has been assembled to provide some idea of Freud's thinking about lesionless pain over the period 1884–1895. From Anna O.'s persistent facial pain and the complications of drug treatment for chronic pain, to debates about conversion and the ideogenesis of pain and finally to the equivocation between *schmerz* and *unlust*, the evidence all points to the central place of pain without lesion in the origins of psychoanalytic theory and practice.

## Notes

1. Tuke, 1872, *Illustrations of the influence of the mind upon the body in health and disease designed to elucidate the action of the imagination.*
2. *Ibid.*, ix–xi.
3. *Ibid.*, 29.
4. *Ibid.*, 34.
5. *Ibid.*, 55.
6. *Ibid.*, 124–5.
7. Clark, 1981, 301, *The rejection of psychological approaches to mental disorder in late nineteenth-century British psychiatry.*
8. Beveridge, 1991, *Thomas Clouston and the Edinburgh School of Psychiatry.*
9. Clouston, 1883, *Clinical Lectures on Mental Diseases.*
10. Clouston, 1886, *The relationship of bodily and mental pain.*
11. Meynert, 1884, *Psychiatry: a clinical treatise on diseases of the fore-brain.*
12. Clark, 1981, *The rejection of psychological approaches to mental disorder in late nineteenth-century British psychiatry.*

13. Sulloway, 1992, 69, *Freud, biologist of the mind: beyond the psychoanalytic legend.*
14. Freud & Breuer, 1895, *Studies on hysteria.*
15. Freud, 1894, *Project for a scientific psychology.*
16. Freud, 1924, *The economic problem of masochism.*
17. David-Ménard, 1989, 66, *Hysteria from Freud to Lacan: body and language in psychoanalysis.*
18. Sulloway, 1992, 24, *Freud, biologist of the mind: beyond the psychoanalytic legend.*
19. Hirschmüller, 1989, 101–16, *The life and work of Josef Breuer: physiology and psychoanalysis.*
20. Sulloway, 1992, 26–8, *Freud, biologist of the mind: beyond the psychoanalytic legend.*
21. Freud, 1900, 111–15, *The interpretation of dreams.*
22. Sulloway, 1992, 35–42, *Freud, biologist of the mind: beyond the psychoanalytic legend.*
23. Freud & Breuer, 1895, *Studies on hysteria.*
24. Sulloway, 1992, ch 3, *Freud, biologist of the mind: beyond the psychoanalytic legend.*
25. Hirschmüller, 1989, 183–6, *The life and work of Josef Breuer: physiology and psychoanalysis.*
26. Freud & Breuer 1895, 135, *Studies on hysteria.*
27. *Ibid.*, 137.
28. *Ibid.*, 157.
29. *Ibid.*, 166.
30. *Ibid.*, 174.
31. *Ibid.*, 178.
32. *Ibid.*, 179.
33. David-Ménard, 1989, ch 1, *Hysteria from Freud to Lacan: body and language in psychoanalysis.*
34. *Ibid.*, 27.
35. Freud & Breuer, 1895, 190, *Studies on hysteria.*
36. Freud, 1900, 104–121, *The interpretation of dreams.*
37. Lacan J, 1988, ch 13 and 14, *Seminar II: The Ego in Freud's Theory and in the technique of Psychoanalysis.*
38. Freud, 1894, *Project for a scientific psychology.*
39. Knight, 1984, *Freud's project: a theory for Studies on Hysteria.*
40. Levin, 1978, ch 7, *Freud's early psychology of the neuroses: a historical perspective.*
41. Sulloway, 1992, 113–31, *Freud, biologist of the mind: beyond the psychoanalytic legend.*

# 8

## Pain as Psychopathology in early twentieth-century French and German Psychiatric Writings: 1900–1914

It is tempting to end this history of responses to the problem of pain without lesion with Freud's famous articulation of hysterical conversion. But it would be wrong to do so for at least three reasons. Firstly, it is historiographically weak since it inevitably implies that all the material in Chapters One to Six was a 'prehistory' of psychoanalysis. This tempts the reader to focus on issues of precedence and overstates the impact of psychoanalysis on the clinical practice of psychiatry in our own century, especially in Britain. Secondly, and more importantly, it blinds us to the fact that it was someone else entirely who coined the term 'psychogenic pain', emphasized the wide range of psychological influences on the genesis of pain and drew a crucial, but now forgotten, distinction between psychogenic and ideogenic pain. This was Otto Binswanger in his monumental 1904 textbook on hysteria. Thirdly, ending the account with Freud on hysterical pain would exclude a fascinating discussion among French alienists about lesionless pain in a number of other mental disorders, culminating in an extraordinary text by Blondel in which the relationship between pain as an experience and pain language was most fully considered.

### 1. Otto Binswanger on Psychogenic Pain.

Professor Otto Binswanger of Jena [1852–1929] was the uncle of the much better known Ludwig Binswanger, the Swiss psychiatrist who worked with Jung at the Burghölzi, travelled with him to meet Freud in 1907 and later became Director at Bellevue, Kreuzlingen and a leading psychoanalyst.[1] Otto was an earlier member of the 'Binswanger dynasty' who directed the asylum in Jena and wrote a standard psychiatric text on hysteria, *Die Hysterie* in 1904[2]. 660 pages of this 950 page monograph were devoted to the symptomatology of hysteria but I shall offer an exposition of just 13 pages on pain.

Binswanger begins by siding with Erb and against von Frey. He states:

> it is our daily experience that sensations of pain are subject to wide

171

individual variation which cannot be explained in terms of varying
excitation of a terminal apparatus of peripheral nerves [i.e. von Frey's
'pain spots'].

Rather he follows Weber, Erb and others in arguing that 'pain is
only a special kind of negative intonation of feeling/sensation
[*Gefühl*] related to the stimulation of centripetally conducting
nerves'.[3] Pain intensity is a function of stimulus intensity or of the
state of excitation (or 'psychic receptivity') of the central nervous
substance for pain.

He then describes two sorts of hyperalgesia. One stems from
pathological peripheral stimulation. Inflammatory pain is the
example chosen. The other, psychical hyperalgesia *[psychische
hyperalgesie]*, arises from a pathological alteration of psychic
processes. From a physiological viewpoint an increase in excitation or
a decrease in inhibition in the cortical sensory cells is at play. From a
psychical perspective the result is increased pain sensation.
Binswanger emphasizes the overriding importance of 'higher' cortical
or psychic influences over mere peripheral factors with a case history.[4]
He describes a female patient with a 'circular affective psychosis' who
also happened to suffer tuberculosis of the thoracic spine. She felt no
pain during manic phases, bearable pain when in a normal mood
state and very severe pain, relieved only by morphine, when
depressed: 'without doubt the pathological mood has been the
decisive factor for the sensation of pain'.

Binswanger now expounds the case for the importance of mood
in the genesis of localized bodily pain in patients suffering hysteria.
'Psychic pain can present with a defined eccentric projection without
local lesion'[5] but he felt the term 'ideogenic pain' was not quite right
to express this.

> There is no need for the appearance of an idea [*Vorstellung*] of a
> particular disease or for the concentration of attention on certain
> physical conditions to provoke such pains: a disturbance of mood
> suffices, which causes localised sensations of pain via
> irradiation...Therefore one would prefer the term 'psychogenic pain'
> for these pains.[6]

Thus Binswanger emphasized that low mood is at least as
important a cause of local pain without lesion as the patient's ideas
that Freud had drawn attention to. This broad meaning of
psychogenic pain has been lost over the course of the twentieth
century and most psychiatrists reserve the term 'psychogenic' for

cases where ideogenesis seems to have occurred. In cases where depressed mood may account for lesionless pain a diagnosis of a depressive illness is now made. Thus we do seem to have lost sight of a continuous line of thought that ran from Griesinger via Meynert to Binswanger. All these authors favoured a Romantic monist theory of pain which emphasized the radical equivalence of non-localized pain of melancholia and the localized lesionless pain of certain neuroses.

### 2. *Les Douleurs Psychopathiques –* Psychopathologies of Pain in French Psychiatric Writings 1907–1914.

In a 1907 article in the influential journal *L'Encephale* entitled 'Les Cénestopathies'[7] Dupré & Camus revived the view that some lesionless pain arose from disordered bodily sensation or cenesthesis. Their paper began thus:

> *Nous proposons de désigner sous le nom de Cénestopathies les altérations de la sensibilité commune ou interne, c'est-à-dire les troubles de ces sensations qui incessamment arrivent au cerveau de tous les points du corps et qui, à l'état normal, ne s'imposent à notre attention par aucun caractère particulier, soit dans leur intensité, soit dans leur modalité. On sait de quelle importance est ce domaine de la cénesthésie, le fondement primitif de notre personnalité. On connaît aussi la fréquence, la variété et le rôle majeur de ces troubles au cours des différentes affections mentales.*
>
> *Chez certains sujets, ces malaises sensitifs, par leur existence unique ou hautement prépondérante dans le tableau clinique, par leur intensité, par leur persistance, par leur caractère spécifique et leur évolution dégagée de tout autre syndrome, acquièrent un intérêt théorique et practique de premier ordre...*
>
> *Il se présente fréquemment, aux consultations de Neurologie et de Psychiatrie, des malades qui se plaignent d'éprouver, dans différentes parties du corps, des sensations anormales, généralement douloureuses, mais toujours pénibles et étranges, dont la durée persistante les affecte et dont la nature insolite les trouble et les inquiète.*
>
> *Ces malades souffrent avant tout de troubles de la sensibilité interne...*

The text goes on to state that personal idiosyncratic reactions to these sensory disturbances cloud the clinical picture and often lead to misdiagnosis as anxiety, hypochondria or a delusional state.

Dupré & Camus gave six case histories to establish this new syndrome. I shall present just three:

CASE 1. A 48-year-old Jew of high intelligence. The only son of a nervous mother. Digestive tract symptoms throughout his twenties, notably stomach pain associated with headache. At 30, after a period of sleep deprivation and sexual excess, new symptoms arose: violent head pain, spasms of the pharynx and oesophagus. He stopped work and made numerous medical consultations over the next 18 years. When seen by the authors his symptoms included a feeling that his brain was atrophied, 'like a sponge', and insensibility of the whole oral cavity. On examination he was noted to repeatedly put his fingers in his mouth to confirm the insensibility and to pinch, pick and scratch at his face. Memory, judgement, association of ideas, moral sensibility and affectivity were all preserved. Physical examination revealed no lesion. *'L'examen objectif de la sensibilité dénote une hyperesthésie généralisée'.*

CASE 2. A 39 year-old woman, with a tuberculous father and an alcoholic mother who had died of cirrhosis. Alcoholic grandparents. A sister who was an *idiote* interned in a hospital and a brother who died of tuberculosis. The patient had been ill for years with multiple hospitalizations. She had a number of symptoms, mostly around the head: a sensation of painful pulling of the nerves behind her ears, traction inside her eyes and nasal canal, a sensation of emptiness inside her head and eyes, of displacement of all intracephalic organs, of balls rolling along *'des gouttières carotidiennes'.* Also pains in the throat, heart and back. She had formulated suicide plans because of this permanent state. Physical examination was normal: *'La sensibilité objective, superficielle et profonde, semble partout normale'.*

CASE 5. An 18 year-old Russian Jew – 'unstable psychopath'. Mother, two brothers and a sister all constantly ill. Father tuberculous. Patient had been prone to tiredness and headache since infancy. Complains of constant headache, weakness and fatigue as well as pains in the chest and abdomen.

> *Ces douleurs n'affectant pas aucun territoire anatomique ni fonctionnel spécial, elles sont de nature imprécise, elles s'accompagnent d'une sensation de lourdeur vague, de gêne pénible dans la profondeur, de souffrance générale et diffusée à tous les organes et à tous les tissus.*

Examination revealed no lesion and no stigmata of hysteria except for a hint of right-sided hyperaesthesia. The exclusion of a primary diagnosis of hysteria was obviously necessary if the proposed new diagnosis of cenestopathy was to be sustained.

In a discussion of the differential diagnosis of their new syndrome, the authors devoted most space to hysteria and neurasthenia (which they discussed together as hystero-neurasthenia) and hypochondria. They argued that most lesionless pain fell into the category of hystero-neurasthenia. Such neurotics complained specifically of straightforward pains in various parts of the body, while cenestopaths complained of poorly localized sensory disturbances more alarming and more distressing than mere pain. Secondly, the pain in hystero-neurasthenia evolved in relation to the general health of the patient and was readily modified by analgesics, emotions, suggestion and psychotherapy. None of this was true for the symptoms of cenestopathy. Thus it is clear that these authors were trying to capture a more generalized and profound disturbance of the relationship between a subject and his body.

The differential diagnosis with hypochondria was also rather subtle. Hypochondriacs misinterpreted their bodies and built systematized pathological beliefs around their symptoms which they held very firmly. They developed strong views about the origins of their physical disorder. By contrast, cenestopaths experienced their bodies in an unusual way and struggled to express these feelings in words. They did not elaborate or systematise their beliefs about the problem or its origin. While hypochondriacs resigned themselves to their gloomy situation and abandoned their social lives in favour of introspection, cenestopaths maintained hope of a cure and tried to live on.

By the time of the 1911 Congress of French Alienists and Neurologists at Amiens, Maillard was drawing clear distinctions between four types of psychopathological pain: disordered cenesthesia, hysterical somatic symptom, somatic hallucination and hypochondriacal delusion.[8] The language in which the patient described his pain held the key to the difficult differential diagnosis between them.

Maillard began by asserting that pain consists essentially of a modification of cenesthesis, where cenesthesis is the common feeling of all internal and external sensations ('*sentiment commun à toutes nos sensations internes ou externes*'). He drew a distinction between physiological pain and psychopathological pain (*douleur psychopathique*). This latter was a symptom of an abnormal mental state and not dependent upon any organic lesion. Four categories of such psychopathological pain were then proposed:

1. *HALLUCINATORY PAIN* – classically to be found in states of intoxication and systematized persecutory delusional states. The distinction between such an hallucination and hypochondriacal misinterpretation of the condition of one's own body hinged on the objective character and fleeting duration of hallucinatory pain as opposed to the very chronic persistence of hypochondriacal beliefs and their highly subjective expression in language.

2. *DOULEURS PITHIATIQUES* – arising from hysterical autosuggestion, typically after an occupational accident of some sort. A disorder of attention, governed by desire or dread, lay at the root of such pain. It became a sort of *idée fixe.* These pains could be recognized clinically by exaggeration and discordance in the patients' reactions and by their susceptibility to suggestion. This category of pains would undoubtedly have been dubbed 'hysterical pain' a few years earlier, and indeed Dupré & Camus had accepted that denomination in 1907. Maillard's preference for 'pithiatism' betrays the influence of Babinski's attack on Charcot's work on hysteria. Babinski drew attention to the centrality of suggestion in the genesis of hysterical phenomena and renamed the condition to reflect this new emphasis. Maillard's reference to an *idée fixe* was no doubt a nod towards Janet's work. For discussion of these post-Charcotian developments in France see Noel Evans.[9]

3. *PARANOIAC PAIN* – caused by delusional misinterpretation of mundane, non-painful bodily sensations (e.g. tiredness, fullness, shivering). This pain was governed by a delusional belief, typically a hypochondriacal or zoopathic delusion.

4. *CENESTOPATHIC PAIN* – as described by Dupré & Camus.

In the discussion that followed Maillard's presentation, Charles Blondel asked at what point the struggle to verbalize the odd sensations of the cenestopath ended and the linguistic elaboration and systematization of delusional belief of the hypochondriac began? It is to his writings, which explore the relation between language and lived experience in some depth, that we must turn to conclude this chapter.

Blondel's *La Conscience Morbide* of 1914[10] develops an argument that can only be well understood in the light of the material presented already here. The book has had negligible influence on Anglophone psychiatry but was of importance to French psychiatrists of the 1920s, among them Jacques Lacan. Lacan was still referencing Blondel in his seminars of the mid-1950s. *La Conscience Morbide* is of considerable interest to the history of pain without lesion because it addresses at some length the relationship between pain as a private experience and pain language.

Blondel started with the observation, inspired, he says, by Durkheim, that 'we do not create our language'. Rather it is a collective or social phenomenon, imposed from without, that provides the conceptual apparatus by which we organize even our most private thoughts. Our use of this language, be it in thought or speech, purges our experience of all its singular or idiosyncratic elements, leaving only that which can be shared. In a nutshell, language achieves the 'subordination of our individual states to concepts'. Cenesthesis, the most private, personal and fundamental lived experience of all, is inexpressible and escapes language. This is of no consequence in the healthy since cenesthesis is a dimly perceived foundation on which more interesting perception of the external world is based. Occasionally 'normals' get a headache but they do not become insane trying to precisely describe the unique aspects of this experience:

> [When a pain] stands out more acutely from the cenesthetic mass, it is only by a series of artifices that we can form any idea of it. We localise it; we compare it to such and such a sensory impression as a prick, a burn, or a feeling of pressure; we enquire into its causes....We are satisfied with this notation. And yet it only circumscribes our pain without representing it! Without this notation we could say nothing about the pain, and even with it there remains something which cannot be expressed. But – and this is the essential point – the normal individual is not concerned about what this inexpressible element in his pain may be.[11]

Thus 'normals' turn away from 'unique mental states'. This can be assisted by good socialization – 'coming back amongst men'.[12]

In madness there is no change in the nature of cenesthesis, it simply comes to attention and the patient 'loses himself in futile search for a discursive system which would be more closely wedded to the form of his thoughts and feelings'.[13] Thus:

> Cenesthesia plays a fundamental part in the genesis of certain mental illnesses. But in order to play this part it has no need to undergo any intrinsic modification. All it need do...is to rise in all its obscure presence and restore to the sound mind the indistinctness,...the irreducible originality of what is purely psychological and essentially individual.[14]

177

Blondel argued against disordered cenesthesis, opposing Dupré & Camus, in the genesis of mental illness.

Blondel gave a number of case histories, notably one Adrienne who used a wealth of images and metaphors to express her hypochondriacal preoccupations. Dupré & Camus had supposed that a disturbance of cenesthesis was the primary pathology in such a case and the language phenomena secondary. Blondel accepted that many of the asylum patients he had listened to, in some cases for years, did employ the same form of words as 'normals' might if they had a pain:

> Undoubtedly some of our patients make certain complaints almost identical with those we ourselves make; it seems difficult, therefore, not to admit behind them pains at least analogous to ours. Migraine, headaches...intercostal neuralgia, cramp, tinglings, prickings.. .rheumatism; pains in the forehead, the gums, the back of the neck, the throat, arms, chest, loins, stomach, knees, feet and ankles... such is a list of symptoms in Adrienne [and other patients].[15]

They do often use the same metaphors that we might choose: 'an iron bar...pressure...heaviness... a knife... a hook...a cord being tightened... lightening'. However these metaphors, when used by the patients, are 'double-faced': on one side they are understandable efforts to verbalize cenesthesis, on the other they form part of a delusional system. This can only be discerned by the most careful listening clinician. For example, a patient named Gabrielle suffered abdominal pains without lesion and had a delusion of pregnancy. Most clinicians, Blondel asserted, would think it obvious that the delusion was secondary to the pain, an effort to make sense of the cenesthetic sensation. But the patient herself commented that the abdominal pains did not resemble the pains of a previous pregnancy as she remembered them and Blondel therefore concluded that the delusion of pregnancy, that is, a disturbance of belief expressed in language, was primary in this case. He made two further arguments against a primary disturbance of cenesthesis in psychotic cases of pain without lesion. When there happens to be an organic or functional lesion these patients tend to ignore it if anything. For example, Adrienne had inflamed fallopian tubes but no symptom from these figured among her many pain complaints. Finally, Blondel drew attention to the hypertrophy of metaphorical language, the 'frenzy of interpretation' encountered in these patients as opposed to the brief verbalizations of a 'normal' who may say 'I've got a crashing headache' but is unlikely to spend months and years struggling to find the right words. This hypertrophy of language was the primary mental state abnormality for Blondel.

It is important to clarify the patient group Blondel was writing about. He emphasized that he was describing lesionless pain among asylum inpatients. His conclusion was that for many of them pain was secondary to a delusional system and a disturbance of belief and language was primary. Dupré & Camus, in contrast, had argued for a primary disturbance of bodily feeling in at least one interesting subgroup of patients with lesionless pain.

What I hope to have made clear in this brief glance at a rather 'alien' alienist literature is the way the speech of the pain patient came to be of paramount importance to certain French psychiatrists a generation before Freudian psychoanalysis penetrated that country. I have also drawn attention to descriptions of a number of psychopathologies of pain besides that of hysterical conversion.

## Summary

In this chapter we have seen how the Continental psychiatric literature of the early twentieth century included a complex and nuanced approach to pain without lesion. The role of suggestion, memory, ideas and mood in the genesis of hysterical pain was elucidated and a valuable distinction between ideogenic and psychogenic pain drawn. French alienists became intrigued by the pain complaints of non-hysterical patients and struggled to differentiate between the hypochondriacal delusions of the insane and the bizarre bodily feelings of 'cenestopaths'.

This psychopathology of pain could only be unravelled through listening attentively to the speech of the patient. An argument was developing as to the status of this speech. Did it offer a report of the private pain experience of the individual or was a disturbance of language at the core of the problem of pain without lesion? Either way, the patient's account of their pain had a new importance. This was not a return to the eighteenth-century relationship between physician and patron but the inclusion of speech in an extended medical gaze. The pain patient's use of metaphor was now beginning to attract almost as much medical interest as the condition of the tissues of his body.

## Notes

1. Jones, 1955, *Sigmund Freud: life and work, Volume II.*
2. Binswanger, 1904, *Die Hysterie.*
3. *Ibid.*, 117.
4. *Ibid.*, 119.
5. *Ibid.*, 123.
6. *Ibid.*

7. Dupré & Camus, 1907, *Les Cénestopathies.*
8. Maillard (1911), *Des différent espèces de douleurs psychopathiques: Congrès des aliénistes et neurologistes de France, Amiens.*
9. Noel Evans, 1991, *Fits and starts.*
10. Blondel, 1914, *La conscience morbide.*
11. *Ibid.*, 49–50.
12. *Ibid.*, 52.
13. *Ibid.*, 57.
14. *Ibid.*, 63.
15. *Ibid.*, 77–8.

## Conclusions

### 1. The History of Sensory Examination

Before summarizing the main historical conclusions and their contemporary relevance I should like to draw together the findings of a subplot that has run through the preceding chapters – the changes in bedside examination of chronic pain patients over the course of the century. This is important since any history of ideas that cannot demonstrate any tangible influence of those ideas on practice is weakened. The traditional historiography[1-3] tells us that there was no neurological bedside examination before about 1870 and no meaningful sensory examination until the 1890s. It is argued that 'analytic', as opposed to 'descriptive', sensory examination was impossible until detailed studies of patients with syringomyelia and Brown-Séquard syndrome had clarified the crossed afferent tract for pain in the spinal cord, and vibration and joint position sense had been recognised as indicators of dorsal column integrity. My findings from the case histories of chronic pain patients offer a fuller picture of what sort of 'descriptive' examinations were made earlier in the century.

In the first three decades of the nineteenth century it seems that much of the examination was devoted to establishing the presence or absence of inflammation. By the 1830s attention had switched to examination of the 'spine'. A new clinical sign, Players spots (areas of spinal tenderness), was sought in cases of chronic pain. For example, Teale, Brodie and Swan all applied pressure to the spinal column during bedside examination, the latter percussing with a key. Once again, clinical practice closely followed theoretical innovations – in this case the spinal irritation literature spawned by the Bell–Magendie debate about the spinal nerve roots. Brodie's examinations went further. He looked for oedema, muscle wasting, joint deformity and compared the effects of pinching the skin over a joint with weightbearing. Hyperaesthetic skin over a painful joint became known as Brodie's sign and was used by Charcot in the 1880s as evidence for local hysteria rather than joint disease.

Weber distinguished touch from pain and showed how two-point

181

discrimination varied over the surface of the body. In the 1840s Romberg incorporated these developments in his sensory examinations. In addition, he and Laycock began to systematically compare sensation on the left and right sides of the face and body. This interest in lateralization predated any understanding of decussation of sensory tracts by some 15 years. The writings of Briquet and Handfield-Jones reveal that pressure, pinch, pinprick, electric currents and currents of air were all stimuli applied to the skin of chronic pain patients in routine clinical practice of the 1850s and 1860s. Brown-Séquard lectured on decussation as early as 1858 and argued that touch, pain and temperature were anatomically distinct within the spinal cord but his research did not form the basis of an 'analytic' sensory examination until Charcot's heyday in the 1870s. Now loss of pain sensation, as opposed to touch or temperature, could be interpreted and such distinctions used to localize a neurological lesion, be it functional or structural. The regional distribution of sensory changes took on a new importance once Charcot had noted the 'glove and stocking' pattern in hysteria. Now bedside sensory mapping held the key to discriminating ideogenic and neurogenic disorders. By the time of Gowers's *Manual* the differing localizing significance of anaesthesia, analgesia, hyperaesthesia and hyperalgesia was quite well understood. Therefore I would argue that a 'mature' analytic sensory examination was possible from the late 1880s onwards.

By the 1880s the clinical examination of the pain patient had a further new dimension. The language they used to describe their pain had come under scrutiny and was seen as an important sign that could be used to distinguish between neurosis and insanity. In Allbutt's writings on neuralgic and hysterical neurotics we see material that would nowadays figure in the 'appearance and behaviour' section of a mental state examination used in the differential diagnosis. In the early twentieth century the mental state examination of the chronic pain sufferer was placed alongside reports of neurological examination in the writings of Dupré & Camus, Maillard and Blondel while Freud tried to discover the meaning of lesionless pains in the context of detailed biographical exploration. So by the end of our period the 'medical gaze' had extended to include pain language as well as pathological lesion.

## 2. Historical Conclusions

The first important lesson from this research is that the history of certain 'psychiatric disorders' is almost exclusively to be found in non-psychiatric clinical settings and texts. This is particularly the case for neurotic conditions. Historical studies confined to psychiatric settings and authors will be highly insensitive to theory and practice concerning non-psychotic patients. So historians of psychiatry should read widely in the history of medicine and surgery.

The problem of pain without structural lesion came to the fore around 1800. In Chapter One I have argued that this problem was a result of Bichat's physiological and pathological research. He used pain as a tool of analysis to discriminate one tissue system from another and, as Foucault has argued, welded disease to the body with the expectation that local symptoms meant localized lesions. Pain, rather than being a disease in its own right as it was for De Sauvages, now became a symptom that pointed to something more fundamental – pathology. Pinel immediately redefined Cullen's neuroses in terms of symptoms lacking structural lesions and the problem of pain without lesion was created. It was continuously tackled in elite medical writings throughout the nineteenth century. Physicians and surgeons responded in the early decades by reviewing the spatial relationship between pain and lesion and by greatly enlarging the concept of lesion. We have seen in Chapter Two how Broussais's concept of a functional lesion, irritation, was widely taken up and probably saved the anatomo-clinical paradigm. A growing knowledge of neuroanatomy and neurophysiology was brought to bear on traditional sympathies. The processes of reflexion, irradiation and eccentricity were used to explain pain at a distance from lesion, as described in Chapter Four. Structural lesions came to be thought of as the appearance resulting from invisible pathological processes. Functional lesions were initially speculative but later became demonstrable in the laboratory and clinic, as in the work of Bernard and Brown-Séquard outlined in Chapter Five. Meanwhile there was an important German Romantic tradition that saw pain as a very different phenomenon than touch or the special senses. In contrast to the Anglo-French emphasis on pain as a marker of lesion, Müller and his followers emphasized the radical physiological equivalence of subjective pain and pain due to pathology. This literature was described in Chapter Three.

In the second half of the century neurologists and psychiatrists drew important distinctions between neuralgic, hysterical, neurogenic, ideogenic and psychogenic pain. At various moments chronic pain without lesion was characterized as an hallucination, an illusion, a delusion, depressed mood or disordered cenesthesis. Russell Reynolds's important distinction between neurogenic and ideogenic pain was described in Chapter Five and Charcot's considerable elaboration of this seminal idea was covered in Chapter Six, along with Clifford Allbutt's efforts to separate neuralgic neurotics from degenerate hysterics. Griesinger's view that chronic pain and melancholia were physiologically identical was later elaborated by Meynert and Clouston as shown in Chapter Seven. The crucial importance of this idea in the genesis of Freud's concept of conversion was also covered there. In Chapter Eight we saw how a useful, but now forgotten, distinction between psychogenic and ideogenic pain was proposed in 1904. Finally the various psychopathologies of pain recognized by French alienists of the early twentieth century were outlined, including an extraordinary meditation on the relationship between pain and language by Blondel.

In Kuhnian terms the history of chronic pain traversed two scientific revolutions in the nineteenth century. The first, around 1800, was the birth of an anatomoclinical method that insisted pain symptoms should have corresponding pathological lesions. The second, in the 1890s, was the novel psychoanalytic method that saw pain complaints as metaphors that could be interpreted in terms of the individual's autobiography. Far from a passive exposure to these changing trends in medical theory I have argued that pain had a central place in driving both these revolutions. Pain was the analytical tool Bichat used to distinguish one tissue from another, and, more crucially, pain was the property of living matter that gave rise to the very concept of tissue systems. And a decade of rather anxious consideration of the causes and management of chronic pain led Freud to theoretical and technical innovations, notably conversion and free association, central to the new discipline of psychoanalysis.

The terms used to name the clinical phenomenon of chronic pain without lesion varied very widely over the course of the century. An abbreviated list would include: sympathetic pain, neuralgia, hysteria, local hysteria, hypochondria, spinal irritation, railway spine, neurasthenic pain, hystero-neurasthenia, ideogenic pain, psychogenic pain and cenestopathic pain.

The primary material gathered in this thesis constitutes a considerable weight of evidence against the historical orthodoxy that the growth of neuroscience in the nineteenth century obscured consideration of the psychological dimensions of pain and rendered pain either 'organic' or 'imaginary'.

The clinical features of pains without structural lesion have displayed some historical invariance despite the fact that both neurogenic and psychogenic pains are mixed within this category (along with some patients in whom structural pathology could be found using modern investigative techniques). Case histories repeatedly refer to continuous, severe, chronic pain complicated by great disability, and often by opiate dependence, but with negligible mortality. The left-sided predominance of lesionless pain is mentioned time and again. This rather static clinical picture speaks against a social constructionist history of lesionless symptoms.

### 3. Contemporary Relevance

It is always risky to specify the relevance of rather pure scholarship in one discipline to another, in this case of history of medicine to contemporary psychiatry. Any relevance, and there may be none, emerges when those with a greater expertise in the second discipline read work in the first. With this caveat in mind I should like to touch upon one or two possible points of contact.

I mentioned in the introduction that contemporary psychiatric nosology of chronic pain without lesion is problematic. Murphy[4] made an excellent critique of the DSM III-R category of Somatoform Pain Disorder.[5] The diagnostic criteria made it clear that this was a diagnosis of exclusion – chronic pain without lesion. Murphy complained that it named a problem not a psychiatric syndrome, and pointed out that no psychopathology whatsoever was specified for this disorder. It thus seemed extremely unclear in what sense Somatoform Pain Disorder was a mental disorder. In the light of my historical research I would add that this diagnosis of exclusion represented a return to the Pinelian definition of neurosis – somatic symptom without lesion – and neglected nearly two hundred years effort to specify the *positive* clinical features of lesionless chronic pain. It effaced the crucial distinction between neurogenic and psychogenic pain and ignored all the physical and mental state abnormalities in chronic pain patients reviewed in this book. A more recent diagnostic category of Pain Disorder (American Psychiatric Association 1994) is defined by the centrality of pain in the clinical presentation and the presence of 'psychological factors...judged to have an important role in the onset, severity, exacerbation, or maintenance of the pain'. Now the presence or absence of lesion is not at issue but the presence of pathogenic or pathoplastic 'psychological factors' is essential. Here the claims for a mental disorder hinge on aetiology and once again phenomenology, be it descriptive or dynamic psychopathology, does not figure. One problem with this category is the failure to distinguish between ideogenic and psychogenic pain. Chronic pain patients with severely depressed mood must be classified as depressed, that is, depression trumps pain disorder in this nosology. Thus any notion that chronic pain and depression may be somehow equivalent or that chronic pain may be caused by depressed mood rather than, say, conflicts or traumatic memories, is written out of this classification. Pain Disorder only covers ideogenic pain but excludes the important tradition of thought, running from Griesinger, via Meynert, to Otto Binswanger, that saw pain and depression as physiologically identical. It is also less than clear why ideogenic pain should be separated from conversion disorder in this nosology.

Two lines of historical continuity identified in my work seem to me to be of heuristic value – the idea of the physiological equivalence of chronic pain and depression and the repeated observation of a left-sided predominance of psychogenic pain. There is some support in contemporary pain research for both. Serotonin depletion is thought to be an important determinant of both depression and chronic pain. Serotonin modulates endogenous opiate secretion and this may be how it influences pain perception.[6] Tricyclic antidepressants are widely used in the management of both neurogenic and psychogenic chronic pain.[7] In a well known paper Blumer & Heilbronn[8] argued for chronic pain as a variant of depression on the basis of several decades of clinical work but both Pilowsky and Merskey insisted that mechanisms of hysterical conversion were more often at play and rejected the idea. Turning to the left-sided predominance of psychogenic pain, highlighted in the contemporary psychiatric literature by Merskey & Watson,[9] it has been argued that this points to a functional lesion of the right hemisphere.[10] There is now a rather wide literature supporting right hemisphere dominance for emotion[11-13] so if chronic pain is physiologically very similar to depressed mood one can see why it might be lateralized.

If there is any substance to the ideas above then the management of chronic pain patients with behavioural psychotherapy, as advocated by Fordyce,[14] is put into question. Ignoring pain complaints and concentrating on tackling inactivity, as widely practised in multidisciplinary pain clinics, may be akin to treating a severely depressed patient behaviourally so as to reduce his verbal complaints and underfunctioning while systematically ignoring his status as a suffering human subject. The target symptoms may be measurably improved while the person in pain is neglected.

## 4. Closing Remarks

This book has been an unashamed history of ideas with the emphasis on elite medical theory, diagnostics and nosology. What might other methodologies, more informed by the social history of medicine, have found? A closer attention to therapeutic practice would have to place the treatment of chronic pain patients in the context of the history of anaesthesia and analgesia, with particular attention to the opiates and cocaine.[15,16] The important gap between the availability and use of treatments for pain is drawn out in Pernick[17]. This gap was largely the result of attitudes to pain and its relief on the part of doctors and patients. The role of the Church in shaping these attitudes was probably more important in France (as described by Rey[18]) than in the United States. Pernick, using quantitative methods in the service of social history, found that only some patients were offered anaesthetics for surgery in North America in the period 1846–1880, despite widespread availability of the techniques. He outlined the judgements made by physicians regarding the sensitivity to pain of women and men, young and old, black and white. Pernick argued that tailoring the dose of anaesthetic according to the individual characteristics of the patient set the doctor apart from the quack with his specifics. Thus what looks to us like rank prejudice once defined medical professionalism. The challenge in writing a history of chronic pain therapeutics would be to match the nuances of this sort of account. A fuller exploration of attitudes to pain might include discussions of corporal punishment, torture and vivisection and would need to span a range of non-medical sources (see Porter[19,20] for overviews of these domains).

Another approach might be a detailed study of certain institutions. On the basis of my research I could commend the University of Berlin in the first four decades of the century or the *Charité* in Paris in the 1840s as likely to be fruitful. This sort of historical writing seeks to establish links between institutional specificity and the ideas emerging from them. An even more localized method is the detailed biographical study of a single historical figure. This allows a much fuller intellectual and personal context from which ideas arise to be provided than has ever been possible in my work. I think Benjamin Brodie and Johannes Müller are two figures who would certainly be worth studying in greater detail with a special focus on their ideas about chronic pain.

I have written a book about a problem very close to the history of hysteria without discussing feminist histories of hysteria, notably the writings of Catherine Clément, Hélène Cixous and Elaine Showalter (see Micale).[21] This omission is for a number of reasons. Firstly, none of them have written about chronic pain as an hysterical symptom. Secondly, the style of the French authors is in part an attempt to escape the conventions of 'phallocentric' academic discourse that makes their work very difficult to respond to (see, for example, Cixous & Clément[22]). Thirdly, I share Micale's view that too much of the historiography of hysteria has been deliberately 'hystericised' and have chosen not to explore the interface between North American literary criticism and French feminist responses to the psychoanalytic thought of Jacques Lacan. Having said this, I am sure it would be possible to make gender the focus of a history of the care of chronic pain patients by male doctors in the nineteenth century. I have drawn attention to the predominance of female chronic pain patients and the theories put up to explain it. I have noted the repeated sensory examinations of the genitalia of patients at the *Charité* by Briquet in the 1850s, the sexualized relationships that Clifford Allbutt and Josef Breuer developed with neuralgic women in 1880, and last, but not least, the enormous influence that Freud's experience with a few women in chronic pain had on his early psychoanalytic thought.

One final approach could be to seek the experience of the patients rather than the doctors. Rey[23] warns that this is likely to be an arduous project because so few bygone sufferers left accounts. Scarry insists that pain's 'resistance to language is not simply one of its incidental or accidental attributes but is essential to what it is.'[24] Despite these problems, sources can be found. For example, Thomas de Quincey's *Confessions of an English Opium Eater*[25] offers a fascinating insight into both his experience of chronic pain and his views concerning its aetiology as well as the effects of opium.

I hope these closing remarks give some idea of the range of work yet to be done on the subject of chronic pain without lesion in the nineteenth century.

### Notes

1. Keele, 1963, *The evolution of clinical methods in medicine.*
2. McHenry, 1969, *Garrison's history of neurology.*
3. Spillane, 1981, *The doctrine of the nerves: chapters in the history of neurology.*
4. Murphy, 1990, *Classification of the somatoform disorders.*
5. DSM III-R, *American Psychiatric Association, 1987.*
6. Feinmann, 1985, *Pain relief by antidepressants: possible modes of*

*action.*

7. Pilowsky & Barrow, 1990, *A controlled study of psychotherapy and amitriptyline used individually and in combination in the treatment of chronic intractable, 'psychogenic' pain.*

8. Blumer & Heilbronn, 1982, *Chronic pain as a variant of depressive disease.*

9. Merskey and Watson, 1979, *The lateralisation of pain.*

10. Trimble, 1989, *Pseudosyndromes.*

11. Gainotti, 1979, *The relationships between emotions and cerebral dominance: a review of clinical and experimental evidence.*

12. Tucker, 1981, *Lateral brain function, emotion and conceptualisation.*

13. Sackheim *et al.*, 1982, *Hemispheric asymmetry in the expression of positive and negative emotions.*

14. Fordyce, 1982, *A behavioural perspective on chronic pain.*

15. Berridge & Edwards, 1981, 62–72, *Opium and the people: opiate use in nineteenth-century England.*

16. Rey, 1993, 155–199, *History of pain.*

17. Pernick, 1985, *A calculus of suffering: pain, professionalism and anaesthesia in nineteenth-century America.*

18. Rey, 1993, 200–5, *History of pain.*

19. Porter, 1993, *Pain and suffering.*

20. Porter, 1994, *Pain and history in the Western World.*

21. Micale, 1995, 66–88, *Approaching hysteria: disease and its interpretations.*

22. Cixous & Clément, 1986, *The newly born woman.*

23. Rey, 1993, 13, *History of pain.*

24. Scarry, 1985, 4, *The body in pain.*

25. Thomas de Quincey, 1822, *Confessions of an English opium-eater.*

# BIBLIOGRAPHY

## Primary Sources:

T. Addison, *Observations on the Disorders of Females Connected with Uterine Irritation* (London: Highley, 1830).

T. C. Allbutt, *On Visceral Neuroses; being the Gulstonian Lectures on Neuralgia of the Stomach and Allied Disorders* (Philadelphia: P. Blakiston, Son & Co., 1884).

F. E. Anstie, *Neuralgia and the Diseases that Resemble it* (London: Macmillan, 1871).

P.-J. Barthez, *Nouveaux Éléments de la Science de l'Homme* (Paris: Goujon & Brunot, 1778).

G. Beard, *A Practical Treatise on Nervous Exhaustion* (New York: William Wood, 1880)

C. Bell, *Essays on the Anatomy of Expression in Painting* (London: Longman, Hurst, Rees & Orme, 1806).
———, *Idea of a new Anatomy of the Brain* (London: Livingstone, 1811). Reprinted in *Sir Charles Bell: His Life and Times*, G. Gordon-Taylor & E. W. Walls (eds), 1958.
———, *The Nervous System of the Human Body* (third edn) (Edinburgh: Adam & Charles Black, 1836).

X. Bichat, *Physiological Researches upon Life and Death* (translated from the second French edition by T. Watkins) (Philadelphia: Smith and Maxwell, 1809).
———, *General Anatomy, applied to Physiology and the Practice of Medicine* (translated from the fifth French edition by C. Coffyn) (London: S. Highley, 1824).

H. Bilon, *Dissertation sur la Douleur* (Paris: Feugueray, 1803).

O. Binswanger, *Die Hysterie* (Vienna: Alfred Hölder, 1904).

R. Blackmore, *A Treatise of the Spleen and Vapours or Hypochondriacal and Hysterical Affections* (London: 1725).

C. Blondel, *The Troubled Conscience and the Insane Mind* (translations from

*La Conscience Morbide* (1914)) (London: Kegan Paul, 1928).

J. Boyle, *A treatise on a modified application of moxa, in the treatment of stiff and contracted joints: and also in chronic rheumatism, rheumatic gout, lumbago, sciatica, indolent tumours, etc, etc.* (second edn) (London: Callow & Wilson, 1826).

P. Briquet, *Traité Clinique et Thérapeutique de l'Hystérie* (Paris: Baillière et fils, 1859).

B. C. Brodie, *Pathological and Surgical Observations on Diseases of the Joints* (London: Longman, Hurst, Rees, Orme & Brown, 1818).
————, *Lectures Illustrative of certain Local Nervous Affections* (London: Longman, Rees, Orme, Brown, Green & Longman, 1837).
————, *Psychological Inquiries* (second edn), (London: Longman, Brown, Breen & Longmans, 1855).

F. J. V. Broussais, *A Treatise on Physiology applied to Pathology* (translated by J. Bell and R. La Roche (Philadelphia: Carey and Lea, 1826).

C. E. Brown-Séquard, *Course of Lectures on the Physiology and Pathology of the Central Nervous System delivered at the Royal College of Surgeons of England in May 1858* (Philadelphia: Collins, 1860).
————, *Lectures on the Diagnosis and Treatment of Functional Nervous Affections* (Cambridge: John Wilson, 1868).

P. J. G. Cabanis, *Rapports du Physique et du Moral de l'Homme* (third edn) (Paris: Caille et Ravier, 1815).

W. B. Carpenter, *Principles of Human Physiology* (fifth edn) (London: J.Churchill, 1855).
————, *Principles of Mental Physiology* (fourth edn) (London: Henry S. King, 1876).

J. M. Charcot, *Lectures on the Diseases of the Nervous System* (translated by G. Sigerson) (London: The New Sydenham Society, 1877).
————, *Clinical Lectures on Diseases of the Nervous System,* Volume III (translated by T. Savill) (London: The New Sydenham Society, 1889).

G. Cheyne, *The English Malady; or a Treatise of Nervous Diseases of all Kinds* (London: 1733).

T. S. Clouston, *Clinical Lectures on Mental Diseases* (London: Churchill, 1883).
————, 'The Relationship of Bodily and Mental Pain', *British Medical Journal* , II (1886), 319–23.

E. Condillac, *Traité des Sensations* (Paris: 1754).

W. Cullen, *Synopsis Nosologiae Methodicae* (Edinburgh: 1769).

J. Darwall, *An Essay on Spinal and Cerebral Irritation* (London: Whittaker, Treacher & Arnot, 1830).

T. De Quincey, *Confessions of an English Opium-Eater* (London: Taylor & Hessey, 1822).

E. Dupré, & P. Camus, 'Les Cénestopathies', *L'Encéphale*, II (1907), 616–31.

W. Erb, *Handbuch der Krankheiten der Peripheren Cerebrospinalen Nerven* (Leipzig: Vogel, 1876).

J. E. Erichsen, *On Concussion of the Spine, Nervous Shock and other Obscure Injuries of the Nervous System* (London: Longmans, Green & Co., 1875).

J. Evans Riadore, *A Treatise on Irritation of the Spinal Nerves* (London: Churchill, 1843).

J. P. Falret, *De l'Hypochondrie et du Suicide* (Paris: Croullebois, 1822).

E. Feuchtersleben, *The Principles of Medical Psychology* (translated by H. Evans Lloyd) (London: Sydenham Society, 1847).

J. G. Fourcade-Prunet, *Maladies Nerveuses des Auteurs, Rapportées à l'irritation de l'Encéphale... avec ou sans Inflammation* (Paris: Delaunay, 1826).

S. Freud, *The Standard Edition of the Complete Psychological Works of Sigmund Freud*, J. Strachey (ed.), (London: The Hogarth Press and the Institute of Psycho-analysis, 1953–74). [SE]
———, *Project for a Scientific Psychology* (1894), in SE I.
———, *The Interpretation of Dreams* (1900), in SE IV.
———, *The Economic Problem of Masochism* (1924), in SE XIX.

S. Freud & J. Breuer, *Studies on Hysteria* (1895), in SE II.

E. J. Georget, *De la Physiologie du Systeme Nerveux, et Spécialement du Cerveau* (Paris: Baillière, 1821).
———, *Recherches sur les Malades Nerveuses en Général, et en Particulier sur le Siège, la Nature et le Traitement de l'Hystérie, de l'Épilepsie et de l'Asthme Convulsif* (Paris: Baillière, 1821).

W. R. Gowers, *A Manual of Diseases of the Nervous System*, Volume I (London: J. & A. Churchill, 1886).
———, *A Manual of Diseases of the Nervous System*, Volume II (London: Churchill, 1888).

# Bibliography

W. Griesinger, *Mental Pathology and Therapeutics* (second edn of 1861) (translated by C. Lockhart Robertson and J. Rutherford) (London: New Sydenham Society, 1867).

C. Handfield-Jones, *Studies on Functional Nervous Disorders* (second edn) (London: John Churchill, 1870).

J. C. Heinroth, *Textbook of Disturbances of Mental Life* (translated and introduced by G.Mora) (Baltimore: Johns Hopkins University Press, 1818 (1975)).

H. von Helmholtz, 'Concerning the Perceptions in General'. An extract from *Physiological Optics* (third edn), in W. Dennis *Readings in the History of Psychology* (New York: Appleton-Century-Crofts, 1948).

J. Hilton, *On the Influence of Mechanical and Physiological Rest in the Treatment of Accidents and Surgical Diseases, and the Diagnostic Value of Pain* (London: Bell & Daldy, 1863).

H. Holland, *Chapters on Mental Physiology* (second edition) (London: Longman, 1858).

T. Laycock, *A Treatise on the Nervous Diseases of Women; Comprising an Inquiry Into the Nature, Causes and Teatment of Spinal and Hysterical Disorders* (London: Longman, Orme, Brown, Green & Longmans, 1840).

M. G. Maillard, 'Des Différente Espèces de Douleurs Psychopathiques: Congrès des Aliénistes et Neurologistes de France, Amiens'. *L'Encéphale,* 6 (1911), 269–82.

J. Marshall, *Practical Observations on Diseases of the Heart, Lungs, Stomach, Liver, etc., etc., occasioned by Spinal Irritation* (Philadelphia: Haswell, Barrington & Haswell, 1837).

T. Meynert, *Psychiatry: a clinical treatise on diseases of the forebrain* (translated by B. Sachs) (New York: Putney, 1885).

J. Müller, *Elements of Physiology* (translated by W. Baly) (London: Taylor & Walton, 1838).

H. W. Page, *Injuries of the Spine and Spinal Cord without apparent Mechanical Lesion, and Nervous Shock, in their Surgical and Medico-legal Aspects* (London: Churchill, 1883).

P. Pinel, *Nosographie Philosophique,* volume II (first edn) (Paris: Caille et Ravier, 1798).
———, *Nosographie Philosophique,* volume III (fifth edn) (Paris: Brossou, 1813).

W. S. Playfair, *The Systematic Treatment of Nerve Prostration and Hysteria* (London: Smith, Elder & Co., 1883)

J. Reid, *Essays on Hypochondriacal and other Nervous Affections* (Philadelphia: Carey & Son, 1817).

M. H. Romberg, *A Manual of the Nervous Diseases of Man*, translated by E. H. Sieveking, (second edn) (London: Sydenham Society, 1853).

J. Russell Reynolds, *The Diagnosis of Diseases of the Brain, Spinal Cord, Nerves and their Appendages* (London: John Churchill, 1855).
————, 'Remarks on Paralysis, and other Disorders of Motion and Sensation, Dependent on Idea', *British Medical Journal* II (1869), 483–5.

C. Scudamore, *A Treatise on the Nature and Cause of Rheumatism with Observations on Rheumatic Neuralgia and on Spasmodic Neuralgia, or Tic Douloureux* (London: Longman, Rees, Orme, Brown & Green, 1827).

F. C. Skey, *Hysteria* (London: Longmans, 1867).

J. Swan, *A Treatise on Diseases and Injuries of the Nerves* (London: Longman, Rees, Orme, Brown, Green & Longman, 1834).
————, *The Brain in Relation to the Mind* (London: Longman, Brown, Green & Longmans, 1854).

G. Tate, *A Treatise on Hysteria* (second edn) (Philadelphia: Carey & Hart, 1831).

T. P. Teale, *A Treatise on Neuralgic Diseases, Dependent upon Irritation of the Spinal Marrow and Ganglia of the Sympathetic Nerve* (Philadelphia: Carey & Hart, 1830).

B. Travers, *An Inquiry Concerning that Disturbed State of the Vital Functions usually Denominated Constitutional Irritation* (New York: Stevenson, 1826).

D. H. Tuke, *Illustrations of the Influence of the Mind upon the Body in Health and Disease Designed to Elucidate the Action of the Imagination* (London: Churchill, 1872).

A. Turnbull, *A Treatise on Painful and Nervous Diseases* (third edn) (London: John Churchill, 1837)

E. H. Weber, *Der Tastsinn und das Gemeingefühl* (translated as *E.H. Weber: The Sense of Touch* by H. E. Ross and D. J. Murray) (London: Academic Press, 1846 (1978)).

R. Whytt, *Observations on the Nature, Causes and Cure of those Diseases which are commonly called Nervous, Hypochondriac or Hysteric; to which are prefixed some Remarks on the Sympathy of the Nerves* (Edinburgh: 1764).

S. Wilks, *Lectures on Diseases of the Nervous System Delivered at Guy's Hospital* (second edition) (London: Churchill, 1883).

## Secondary Sources:

C. Alam & H. Merskey, 'What's in a name? The cycle of change in the meaning of neuralgia', *History of Psychiatry*, 5 (1994), 429–74.

American Psychiatric Association, *Diagnostic and Statistical Manual of Mental Disorders* (third edn, revised) (DSM III-R) (Washington DC: APA, 1987).
———, *Diagnostic and Statistical Manual of Mental Disorders* (fourth edn) (DSM IV) (Washington DC: APA, 1994).

M. J. Aminoff, *Brown-Séquard: a Visionary of Science* (New York: Raven Press, 1993).

C. Bass (ed.), *Somatisation: physical symptoms and psychological illness* (Oxford: Blackwell Scientific Publications, 1990).

H. K. Beecher, *Measurement of Subjective Responses* (Oxford: Oxford University Press, 1959)

V. Berridge & G. Edwards, *Opium and the People: Opiate use in Nineteenth-century England* (London: Allen Lane, 1981).

G. E. Berrios, 'Descriptive psychopathology: Conceptual and Historical aspects', *Psychological Medicine* 14 (1984), 303–13.
———, 'Obsessional disorders during the nineteenth century: terminological and Classificatory issues', in *The Anatomy of Madness*, Volume I, W. F. Bynum, R. Porter & M. Shepherd (eds), (London: Tavistock, 1985).
———, 'Research into the history of psychiatry', in *Research Methods in Psychiatry – a Beginner's Guide*, C. Freeman & P. Tyrer (eds), (second edn) (London: Gaskell, 1992).
———, 'Historiography of Mental Systems and Diseases', *History of Psychiatry*, 5 (1994), 175–190.

G. T. Bettany, *Eminent Doctors: their Lives and their Work* (second edition) (London: John Hogg, 1885).

A. Beveridge, 'Thomas Clouston and the Edinburgh School of Psychiatry', in *150 Years of British Psychiatry, 1841–1991*, G. E. Berrios & H. Freeman (eds), (London: Gaskell, 1991).

D. Blumer & M. Heilbronn, 'Chronic pain as a variant of depressive disease', *Journal of Nervous and Mental Disease*, 170 (1982) 381–411 (includes commentaries by Pilowsky and Merskey).

E. G. Boring, *Sensation and Perception in the History of Experimental Psychology* (New York: Irvington Publishers, 1942)

M. A. Brazier, *A History of Neurophysiology in the 17th and 18th Centuries* (New York: Raven Press, 1984)

G. H. Brown, *Lives of the Fellows of the Royal College of Physicians of London 1826–1925 ('Munk's Roll', Volume IV)* (London: Royal College of Physicians, 1955).

B. Bryan, Wilhelm Erb. Unpublished presentation at Wellcome Institute for the History of Medicine (1994).

M. Budd, *Wittgenstein's Philosophy of Psychology* (London: Routledge, 1989).

W. F. Bynum, 'Varieties of Cartesian experience in early nineteenth-century neurophysiology', in *Philosophical Dimensions of the Neuro-medical Sciences,* Spicker & Engelhardt (eds), (Dordrecht, Holland: Reidel, 1976)
———, 'The nervous patient in eighteenth- and nineteenth-century Britain: the psychiatric origins of British neurology', in *The Anatomy of Madness,* Volume I, W. F. Bynum, R. Porter & M. Shepherd (eds), (London: Tavistock, 1985).
———, *Science and the Practice of Medicine in the Nineteenth Century* (Cambridge: Cambridge University Press, 1994).

G. Canguilhem, *The Normal and the Pathological* (translated by C. R. Fawcett) (New York: Zone Books, 1989).

H. Cixous & C. Clément *The Newly Born Woman* (translated by B. Wing) Manchester: Manchester University Press, 1986).

M. J. Clark, 'Morbid introspection, unsoundness of mind, and British psychological medicine c.1830–c.1900', in *The Anatomy of Madness,* Volume III, W. F. Bynum, R. Porter & M. Shepherd (eds), (London: Routledge, 1988).
———, 'The rejection of psychological approaches to mental disorder in late nineteenth-century British psychiatry', in *Madhouses, Mad Doctors and Madmen: the Social History of Psychiatry in the Victorian*

*Era*, A. Scull (ed.), (London: Athlone Press, 1981).

E. Clarke & L. S. Jacyna, *Nineteenth-century Origins of Neuroscientific Concepts* (London: University of California Press, 1987).

P. F. Cranefield, The organic physics of 1847 and the biophysics of today, *Journal of the History of Medicine and Allied Sciences* 12 (1957) 407–23.

———, *The Way In and the Way Out: François Magendie, Charles Bell and the Roots of the Spinal Nerves* (New York: Futura Pub. Co., 1974).

M. Critchley, *Sir William Gowers 1845–1915: a biographical appreciation* (London: Heinemann, 1949).

M. David-Ménard, *Hysteria from Freud to Lacan: Body and Language in psychoanalysis* (translated by C.Porter) (London: Cornell University Press, 1989).

A. W. Diamond & S. W. Coniam, *The Management of Chronic Pain* (Oxford: Oxford University Press, 1991).

M. Donnelly, *Managing the Mind: a Study of Medical Psychology in early Nineteenth-Century Britain* (London: Tavistock, 1983).

Dowbiggin, I. 'Degeneration and hereditarianism in French mental medicine 1840–90: psychiatric theory as ideological adaptation', in *The Anatomy of Madness,* Volume I, W. F. Bynum, R. Porter & M. Shepherd (eds), (London: Tavistock, 1985).

C. Feinmann, 'Pain relief by antidepressants: possible modes of action', *Pain* 23 (1985) 1–8.

Fischer-Homburger, E. 'Hypochondriasis of the eighteenth century – neurosis of the present century', *Bulletin of the History of Medicine,* XLVI (1972), 391–401.

W. E. Fordyce, 'A behavioural perspective on chronic pain', *British Journal of Clinical Psychology,* 21 (1982) 313–20.

M. Foucault, *The Birth of the Clinic: an Archaeology of Medical Perception* (translated by A. Sheridan) (London: Tavistock Publications, 1973)

R. K. French, *Robert Whytt, the Soul and Medicine* (London: Wellcome Institute Publications, 1969)

G. Gainotti, 'The relationships between emotions and cerebral dominance: a review of clinical and experimental evidence', in *Hemisphere Assymetries of Function in Psychopathology,* J. Gruzelier & P.

Flor-Henry (eds), (Amsterdam: Elsevier, 1979).

T. Gelfand, 'Gestation of the clinic', *Medical History* , 25 (1981) 169–80.

S. L. Gilman, H. King, R. Porter, G. S. Rousseau, & E. Showalter, *Hysteria Beyond Freud* (Berkeley: University of California Press, 1993).

C. C. Gillispie (ed.), *Dictionary of Scientific Biography* (New York: Charles Scribner's Sons, 1970–6).

M. Godet *et al., Dictionnaire Historique et Biographique de la Suisse* (Neuchatel: 1921).

J. Goldstein, *Console and Classify: the French Psychiatric Profession in the Nineteenth Century* (Cambridge: Cambridge University Press, 1987).
———, Empathy as a Category in the Historiography of Psychiatry, Unpublished paper to the Triennial Conference of the European Association for the History of Psychiatry (1993).

F. G. Gosling, *Before Freud: Neurasthenia and the American Medical Community, 1870–1910* (Chicago: University of Illinois Press, 1987).

E. Haigh, *Xavier Bichat and the medical theory of the eighteenth century,* Medical History Supplement 4 (London: Wellcome Institute for the History of Medicine, 1984)

E. Harms, J. C. Reil. *American Journal of Psychiatry,* 116 (1960), 1037–9.

A. Harrington, *Medicine, Mind and the Double Brain* (Princeton, New Jersey: Princeton University Press, 1987).
———, 'Hysteria, hypnosis and the lure of the invisible: the rise of Neo-mesmerism in fin-de-siècle French psychiatry', in *The Anatomy of Madness,* Volume III, W. F. Bynum, R. Porter & M. Shepherd (eds), (London: Routledge, 1988)

R. Harris, 'Murder under hypnosis in the case of Gabrielle Bompard: psychiatry in the courtroom in Belle Époque Paris', in *The Anatomy of Madness,* Volume II W. F. Bynum, R. Porter & M. Shepherd (eds), (London: Tavistock, 1985).

R. Harris, 'Introduction', in *Clinical Lectures on Diseases of the Nervous System* (by J.-M. Charcot), R. Harris (ed.) (London: Tavistock/ Routledge, 1991).

A. Hirschmüller, *The Life and Work of Josef Breuer: Physiology and Psychoanalysis* (London: New York University Press, 1989).

L. S. Jacyna, 'Somatic theories of mind and the interests of medicine in

Britain, 1850–1879' *Medical History*, 26 (1982), 233–58.

———, *Philosophic Whigs: Medicine, Science and Citizenship in Edinburgh, 1789–1848* (London: Routledge, 1994).

———, Alibert, Unpublished paper at the WIHM (1995).

N. D. Jewson, 'The disappearance of the sick man from medical cosmology, 1770–1870', *Sociology*, 10 (1976), 225–44.

E. Jones, *Sigmund Freud: Life and Work,* Volume II (London: The Hogarth Press, 1955).

K. D. Keele, *Anatomies of Pain* (Oxford: Blackwell Scientific Publications, 1957)

———, *The Evolution of Clinical Methods in Medicine* (London: Pitman, 1963).

I. Knight, 'Freud's Project: a Theory for *Studies on Hysteria*', *Journal of the History of the Behavioural Sciences*, 20 (1984), 340–58.

J. Lacan *Seminar II: The Ego in Freud's Theory and in the technique of Psychoanalysis,* translated by S. Tomaselli (Cambridge: Cambridge University Press, 1988).

C. J. Lawrence, *Medicine as Culture: Edinburgh and the Scottish Enlightenment,* unpublished PhD thesis, University of London , 1984.

D. E. Leary, 'Kant, Fichte and Schelling', in *The Problematic Science: Psychology in Nineteenth-century Thought* (eds W. R. Woodward & M. G. Ash) (New York: Praeger, 1982)

———, 'Psyche's muse: the role of metaphor in the history of psychology.' In: *Metaphors in the History of Psychology*, D. E. Leary (ed.), (Cambridge: Cambridge University Press (1990).

S. Lee (ed.), *Dictionary of National Biography* (London: Smith, Elder & Co., 1908–9)

J. E. Lesch, *Science and Medicine in France: the Emergence of Experimental Physiology, 1790–1855* (London: Harvard University Press, 1984).

K. Levin, *Freud's Early Psychology of the Neuroses: a Historical Perspective* (Hassocks, Sussex: The Harvester Press, 1978).

J. M. López Piñero, *Historical Origins of the Concept of Neurosis* (translated by D. Berrios) (Cambridge: Cambridge University Press, 1983).

F. M. Mai & H. Merskey, 'Briquet's *Treatise on Hysteria:* a synopsis and commentary', *Archives of General Psychiatry*, 37 (1980), 1401–5.

O. Marx, 'Nineteenth-century medical psychology: theoretical problems in the work of Griesinger, Meynert and Wernicke', *Isis*, 61 (1970), 355–70.

———, 'German Romantic Psychiatry', Part I, *History of Psychiatry*, 1 (1990) 351–81

R. C. Maulitz, *Morbid Appearances: the Anatomy of Pathology in the early Nineteenth Century* (Cambridge: Cambridge University Press, 1987).

R. Mayou, 'The history of general hospital psychiatry', *British Journal of Psychiatry*, 155 (1989) 764–76.

L. C. McHenry, *Garrison's History of Neurology* (Springfield Illinois: C. C. Thomas, 1969).

D. Mechanic, 'The concept of illness behaviour', *Journal of Chronic Disease*, 15 (1962), 189.

R. Melzack & P. D. Wall, 'Pain mechanisms: a new theory', *Science*, 150 (1965), 971–9.

H. Merskey, *The Analysis of Hysteria* (London: Baillière Tindall, 1979)

———, & F. G. Spear, *Pain: Psychological and Psychiatric Aspects* (London: Baillière, Tindall & Cassell, 1967).

———, & G. D. Watson, 'The lateralisation of pain', *Pain*, 7 (1979), 271–80.

M. S. Micale, 'Hysteria and its historiography: a review of past and present writings', *History of Science*, 27 (1989), 223–61 & 319–51.

———, 'Hysteria and its historiography: the future perspective', *History of Psychiatry*, 1 (1990a) 33–124.

———, 'Charcot and the idea of hysteria in the male: gender, mental science, and medical diagnosis in late nineteenth-century France', *Medical History*, 34 (1990b), 363–411.

———, 'Charcot and *les névroses traumatiques:* historical and scientific reflections', *Revue Neurologique (Paris)*, 150 (1994), 498–505.

———, *Approaching Hysteria: Disease and its Interpretations* (Princeton, New Jersey: Princeton University Press, 1995)

D. B. Morris, *The Culture of Pain* (Berkeley: University of California Press, 1991)

J. Mullan, *Sentiment and Sociability: the Language of Feeling in the Eighteenth Century* (Oxford: Clarendon Press, 1988).

W. Munk, *The Roll of the Royal College of Physicians of London,* Volume III, 1801–25 (London: Royal College of Physicians, 1878)

M. R. Murphy, 'Classification of the somatoform disorders', in *Somatization: Physical Symptoms and Psychological Illness*, C. Bass (ed.), (Oxford: Blackwell Scientific Publications, 1990).

M. Noel Evans, *Fits and Starts: a Genealogy of Hysteria in Modern France.* (London: Cornell University Press, 1991).

M. S. Pernick, *A Calculus of Suffering: Pain, Professionalism and Anaesthesia in Nineteenth-century America* (New York: Columbia University Press, 1985).

I. Pilowsky, 'Abnormal illness behaviour', *British Journal of Medical Psychology,* 42 (1969), 347.
——, & C. G. Barrow, 'A controlled study of psychotherapy and amitriptyline used individually and in combination in the treatment of chronic intractable, "psychogenic" pain', *Pain,* 40 (1990), 3-19.

R. Porter, 'Pain and suffering', in *Companion Encyclopedia of the History of Medicine,* Volume 2, W. F. Bynum & R. Porter (eds), (London: Routledge, 1993).
——, 'Pain and history in the Western World', in *The Puzzle of Pain,* translated by F. Djité-Bruce (Basel: G+B Arts International, 1994).

D. A. Power, *Plarr's Lives of the Fellows of the Royal College of Surgeons of England* (Bristol: John Wright & Sons, 1930).

D. D. Price, *Psychological and Neural Mechanisms of Pain* (New York: Raven Press, 1988).

R. Rey, *History of Pain,* translated by L. E. Wallace, J. A. & S. W. Cadden (Paris: Éditions La Découverte, 1993).

E. H. Reynolds, Structure and function in neurology and psychiatry, *British Journal of Psychiatry,* 157, (1990) 481–90.

G. Rice, 'The Bell–Magendie–Walker Controversy', *Medical History,* 31 (1987), 190–200.

W. Riese & G. E. Arrington, 'The history of J. Müller's doctrine of the specific energies of the senses: original and later versions', *Bulletin of the History of Medicine,* 37 (1963), 179–83.

G. B. Risse, 'Kant, Schelling and the early search for a philosophical science of medicine in Germany', *Journal of the History of Medicine,* 27 (1972), 145–57.
——, 'Schelling, *Naturphilosophie* and John Brown's system of medicine,' *Bulletin of the History of Medicine,* 50 (1976), 321–34.

————, 'Hysteria at the Edinburgh Infirmary: the construction and treatment of a disease, 1770–1800', *Medical History,* 32 (1988), 1–22.

H. D. Rolleston, *The Right Hon. Sir Thomas Clifford Allbutt: a memoir* (London: Macmillan & Co., 1929).

K. E. Rothschuh, *History of Physiology,* translated by G. B. Risse (New York: R. E. Krieger, 1973).

H. A. Sackheim *et al.,* 'Hemispheric assymmetry in the expression of positive and negative emotions', *Archives of Neurology,* 39 (1982), 210–18.

E. Scarry, *The Body in Pain* (Oxford: Oxford University Press, 1985).

F. Schiller, *A Möbius Strip: Fin-de-siècle Neuropsychiatry and Paul Möbius* (Berkeley: University of California Press, 1982).
————, 'Coenesthesis', *Bulletin of the History of Medicine,* 58 (1984), 496–515.

E. Shorter, *From Paralysis to Fatigue: a History of Psychosomatic Illness in the Modern Era* (New York: The Free Press, 1992).

E. Showalter, *The Female Malady: Women, Madness and English Culture 1830–1980* (London: Penguin Books, 1985).

B. Sicherman, 'The uses of a diagnosis: doctors, patients and neurasthenia', *Journal of the History of Medicine and Allied Sciences,* 32 (1977), 33–54.

P. Smith & O. R. Jones, *The Philosophy of Mind* (Cambridge: Cambridge University Press, 1986).

R. Smith, *Inhibition: History and Meaning in the Sciences of Mind and Brain* (London: Free Association Books, 1992).

J. D. Spillane (1981), *The Doctrine of the Nerves: Chapters in the History of Neurology* (Oxford: Oxford University Press, 1981).

J. Starobinski, 'A short history of bodily sensation', *Psychological Medicine,* 20 (1990), 23–33.

M. S. Staum (1980) *Cabanis: Enlightenment and Medical Philosophy in the French Revolution* (Princeton, New Jersey: Princeton University Press, 1980).

F. J. Sulloway, *Freud, Biologist of the Mind: Beyond the Psychoanalytic Legend* (London: Harvard University Press, 1992).

M. R. Trimble, *Post-traumatic Neurosis: from Railway Spine to the Whiplash*

(Chichester: Wiley & Sons, 1981).

————, Pseudosyndromes. Unpublished Sandoz Lecture, Queen Square, 1989.

A. Tuchman, 'Helmholtz and the German medical community', in *H.von Helmholtz and the Foundations of Nineteenth-century Science,* D. Cahan (ed.), (Berkeley: University of California Press, 1993).

D. M. Tucker, 'Lateral brain function, emotion and conceptualisation', *Psychological Bulletin,* 89 (1981), 19–46.

S. Wessely, 'Old wine in new bottles: neurasthenia and "M.E."', *Psychological Medicine,* 20 (1990), 35–53.

S. Wilks, *A Memoir: On the new discoveries or new observations made during the time he was a teacher at Guy's Hospital* (London: Adlard & Son, 1911).

J. P. Williams, 'Psychical research and psychiatry in late Victorian Britain.' In: *The Anatomy of Madness,* Volume I, W. F. Bynum, R. Porter & M. Shepherd (eds), (London: Tavistock, 1985).

L. Wittgenstein, *Philosophical Investigations,* (second edn) (Oxford: Basil Blackwell, 1958).

# Index